the MindB**o**dy FX *life*

MASTERING THE MIND-BODY CONNECTION FOR PERMANENT WEIGHT LOSS

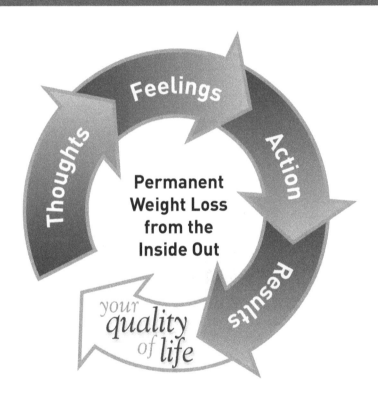

Feelings

Thoughts

Action

Permanent Weight Loss from the Inside Out

Results

your **quality** *of* **life**

MELONIE DODARO

NEW YORK

the MindBody FX
lifestyle

MASTERING THE MIND-BODY CONNECTION FOR PERMANENT WEIGHT LOSS

by Melonie Dodaro
© 2010 Melonie Dodaro. All rights reserved.

ISBN 978-160037-727-3 (paperback)

Library of Congress Control Number: 2009939755

Published by:

MORGAN · JAMES
THE ENTREPRENEURIAL PUBLISHER ™
www.morganjamespublishing.com

Morgan James Publishing
1225 Franklin Ave. Ste 325
Garden City, NY 11530-1693
Toll Free 800-485-4943
www.MorganJamesPublishing.com

Interior Design by:
Bonnie Bushman
bbushman@bresnan.net

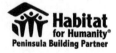

In an effort to support local communities, raise awareness and funds, Morgan James Publishing donates one percent of all book sales for the life of each book to Habitat for Humanity. Get involved today, visit
www.HelpHabitatForHumanity.org.

The information and guidance provided in this book are not intended to be a substitute for medical advice. You should first consult your healthcare practitioner before commencing a new exercise or implementing any suggestions regarding diet, including supplements or herbal or nutritional treatments. The author and publisher expressly disclaim responsibility for any adverse effects arising directly or indirectly from information contained in this book.

Dedication

I dedicate this book to YOU!

May you experience your life at your ideal weight and enjoy all the health, happiness and confidence you deserve.

Acknowledgements

John L. Bigatton, BSc, MSc, MSpSc

John Bigatton is a Strength and Conditioning Coach and Peak Performance Consultant for MindBody FX Weight Management Company. He brings 16 years of experience in fitness and nutrition to the company's team of experts.

Bigatton has consulted for competitive sports teams and top athletes, helping them to achieve high-caliber performances by reprogramming their minds while conditioning the body.

He has developed the "SSS" Training System, a proven method that helps people achieve fat loss by training for as little as 13 minutes a day. This system has been incorporated into The Complete MindBody FX Lifestyle Program.

Angela Wright, BSc, CNP, RNCP

Angela Wright is the creator of The MindBody FX Nutrition Plan for MindBody FX Weight Management Company. At MindBody FX, Wright focuses on helping people take small steps toward making better dietary and lifestyle choices so they can achieve optimum health and emotional wellness.

Wright is a Registered Nutritional Consulting Practitioner (RNCP). She's earned her bachelor's degree with honors in environmental science, and a minor in chemistry and biology

Foreword

For over three decades, I've taught millions of people around the globe how to tap into their unique greatness and maximize their potential.

Melonie Dodaro is an author, weight loss expert, wellness coach and speaker. Her innovative and life-changing approach shows the importance of the power of the mind in improving one's health and well-being.

I've always taught people that the choices you make today will determine the quality of your life in the future, whether you're looking to achieve wealth or health. The great part about this book is it incorporates the importance of the mind-body connection. In order to live your dreams, you need to be living in a healthy body, one that you desire and deserve.

It's apparent that Melonie is a leading authority on weight loss and *The MindBody FX Lifestyle* book has truly found the missing link in the weight loss industry. In this easy to follow, step-by-step process, you'll be shown how to achieve your ideal weight and get off the dieting rollercoaster. This book is one of the best investments that you will ever make in yourself.

— **Les Brown**, Motivational Speaker and Author

Table of Contents

Preparing for Change

Autobiography in Five Short Chapters by Portia Nelson

I. I walk down the street. There is a deep hole in the sidewalk. I fall in. I am lost...I am helpless. It isn't my fault. It takes forever to find a way out.

II. I walk down the same street. There' is a deep hole in the sidewalk. I pretend I don't see it. I fall in again. I can't believe I' am in the same place. But it isn't my fault. It still takes a long time to get out.

III. I walk down the same street. There' is a deep hole in the sidewalk. I see it there. I still fall in...it's a habit. My eyes are open. I know where I am. It' is my fault. I get out immediately.

IV. I walk down the same street. There' is a deep hole in the sidewalk. I walk around it.

V. I walk down another street.

Imagine this street. It's a picturesque street, lined with gorgeous flowering trees whose canopies surround you like a warm sweater. Their scent wafts down around you. The sun is streaming down, warming the pavement under your feet. The breeze is light and soothing. Homes along this street are welcoming. Children are playing and laughing. People you see are smiling and happy. They wave to you. You're standing at one end of the street. At the other end is your ideal weight. You know it's there; you can see it and it seems like an easy stroll down the street toward it, so you start walking. One foot in front of the other...how difficult can it be, you wonder, to reach the end of the street and your ideal weight?

It's a clear path. No worries. One step, then another and another... you stumble on a stone...another step...a car backs out of a driveway and doesn't see you. You stop short. Carry on. Your ideal weight is just over there — easy to get to, you say to yourself. You move forward. There's a sidewalk café...with a tempting aroma coming from inside. A hot, creamy cappuccino and warm pastry would be nice. You sit down. Relax. Enjoy.

It's time to get up now. You linger. It's hard to leave the comfort of the café. In walks Melonie Dodaro. She knows the path to your ideal weight. She beckons you to follow her. Go ahead, and don't look back; Melonie will guide you past the potholes and obstacles along the street and give you the key to unlock the box that holds your desired weight.

You've very likely walked down that street and fallen in the same hole Portia Nelson refers to in her poem — and you've probably done it more than once. We've all started a diet, started walking down that street, and were able to get through a week, maybe even three or four, figuring this was the last time we'd have to diet. Then the dreaded day comes when something just throws you for a loop and you reach automatically for that treat, and then another, and before you know it the box of donuts, bag of candy, or tray of freshly baked cookies has disappeared. Without thinking, you've stuffed temptation into your mouth and started sliding back to your old weight. You're not alone; we've all gone through some version of this scenario. The secret is to figure out why you keep falling in that hole. By reading this book, you've already taken the first step to learning why success has eluded you and how to permanently achieve your ideal weight.

If you have any type of problem—weight, money, relationship or business—understand this: your woes originate from the inside. They originate in the non-physical world and merely manifest in the material world. *The MindBody FX Lifestyle* deals with thoughts and beliefs— the primary cause of all problems. Although this book deals specifically with weight, you'll become aware that the philosophy that builds its foundation can be used to accomplish any goal in your life, from health to wealth.

Welcome. As the CEO and founder of MindBody FX Weight Management Company Inc., I'm so grateful and excited to introduce you to *The MindBody FX Lifestyle*. I'm going to show you to the missing link to weight loss that has eluded you and kept you from achieving your ideal weight.

Have you found yourself wondering why you haven't accomplished the things you desire in your life? For instance, how often have you have tried to reduce your weight? I was in the weight-loss industry for more than a decade as the owner of many weight-loss centers, and I've worked with thousands of clients. Over time, I noticed that clients who had *positive attitudes* and *believed they would achieve success* were always successful at achieving their goal weight. Conversely, clients who made excuses for why they gained weight and had negative thoughts and attitudes (whether they realized it or not), rarely achieved their desired goals. You can't imagine the comments I've heard, starting with statements that begin with "I can't": *I can't eat breakfast; I can't live without my coffee; I can't get up at 6 a.m. to exercise; I can't feed my family this way; I can't seem to lose weight!* You name it…I've heard them all.

My Realization = Your Path to Change

As a long-time student of self-development, I came across the DVD *The Secret* several years ago, and found that I was inspired by its premise—although I did feel it was missing "action," a fundamental key to success. I began to study with some of the top mind potential and human behavior experts, and learned that you attract into your life whatever you give your attention to, whatever you focus on — good or bad. You're made up of energy, which sends out vibrations that range in frequency, based on how you're feeling. For example, when you're going on a vacation, you're excited to go; you feel free from your daily stresses and you get relaxed very quickly. These are good vibrations that lead to a positive state of mind.

Then there are the days you wake up on the wrong side of the bed. You're out of milk. The dog has left you a little reminder that you didn't walk him last night. Traffic is a nightmare; you're running late for work. You spill coffee on your shirt when someone cuts you off. You get to work and your boss wants to see the project you were supposed to finish, and — oh, no! — it's on your kitchen table. Then to top it all off, in walks the customer from your worst nightmare. Nothing is going right. You wonder, why me? What did I do to deserve such a rotten day? Let me tell you…and you may have already guessed that it has something to do with vibrations.

All morning you've been cursing everyone else, feeling sorry for yourself and screaming inside, "why do these things always happen to me?" It's likely that you woke up worrying about your day and have been running various negative thoughts through your mind without even realizing it ever since. Those thoughts are associated with negative vibrations that are sent to your body and to those around you…and they're the reason for your misfortune.

Have you ever been around someone whose negativity you could sense? Did you notice how it affected you? It will usually change how you feel and think. The vibration of thoughts and actions will affect you and those around you.

Once I truly understood this and began to relate these theories to my reality, I realized **what was missing in the weight loss industry was the power of the mind.** That explained why some people were successful and some were not. Just eliminate the words don't, won't, can't, shouldn't, not, and no from your vocabulary and watch what happens. You'll quickly find you can do anything to which you truly commit; it starts with choosing the thoughts that will lead you take the actions necessary to achieve your goals.

Everyone you meet claims to be concerned about health and weight, but few seem to make positive changes. Why? I've seen this problem reach frightening levels...because we focus solely on eating healthy and exercising to achieve our ideal weight. While both those things are important components to a healthy lifestyle, if your mind's not on board, you're wiring yourself to keep falling into that hole.

Stop thinking about what you don't want; start thinking about what you want. Stop avoiding change. Start listening to yourself and to the excuses you use to keep from moving forward toward your dreams and aspirations. You may say things such as "I'm too busy to...; I'd love to, but...; If I were slimmer I'd..." You have to set your mind on your chosen goal and visualize it as though it's already yours — then watch as your dreams come true. When you really believe in something or really want something, you can have it. The only one who's prevented you in the past is you — your own mind. I'm going to show you how to control your mind so you can control your results in life.

Start your journey today toward your ideal weight. Whatever it is, it can be done. When your thoughts turn negative, turn them around. Believe in yourself and your goal and follow the steps outlined in this book.

The Need to Change

It's no secret that we, as a society, are obsessed with diet and weight. Proof of this can be seen every day in the media with the promotions of the latest fad diets featuring slim models from Hollywood and Madison Avenue. You'd think we'd all be fabulously healthy and living life at our ideal weight without a care in the world. However, in a horribly warped contradiction, studies show that U.S. obesity rates have reached epic proportions. What's really going on?

Much of the frustration surrounding our weight loss issues stems from the lies we create, the excuses we give and what we believe. The good news is that it's also within our power to change...and it's becoming more urgent that we do so with each passing day. Just look at these grim statistics:

- Results from the 2003-2004 National Health and Nutrition Examination Survey estimate that 66% of American adults are categorized as either overweight or obese.

- One-third of children and teens between the ages of 2 and 19 are overweight or at risk of becoming so. This has nearly tripled since the 1970s.

- Nearly 78% of Americans are not meeting basic activity level recommendations.

- Approximately 25% of Americans live completely sedentary lives.

- Since 1990, there's been a 76% increase in Type II diabetes in adults 30-40 years old.

- About 300,000 deaths are attributed to obesity each year.

- In 2000, the economic cost of obesity in the U.S. was $117 billion.

The American and Canadian governments, faced with the distressing reality that two-thirds of all Americans and half of all Canadians are overweight or obese, have redesigned their food pyramid guides, hoping to encourage people to eat healthier. Until recently, the food guides placed emphasis on cereals, breads, and other grains; fruits and vegetables; dairy and meats; and fats and oils. The new food pyramid guide recognizes that one size does not fit all, and says you should "make smart choices from every food group…and get the most nutrition out of your calories." In other words, it's best to emphasize "smart choices" such as whole grains, fruit and vegetables, nuts and seeds, and healthy fats, while reducing the intake of sugar, alcohol, red meat, dairy, starchy vegetables, white pasta, and white bread — the foods that often cause weight gain and digestive problems.

How do we stop this ridiculous spiral of poor health and obesity? How do we as a collective consciousness end the madness and stop killing ourselves with the effects of processed food and sedentary lifestyles? Whatever happened to survival of the fittest? If our ancestors had eaten as we do today, a very high percentage of us wouldn't be here.

Studies suggest that for the first time in history, American children's life expectancies are now less than those of their parents. That's not because our medical system is worse, but because of what we feed our children. This is a scary statistic and one that should wake us all up. Stop bringing processed foods into your home! Get your kids moving — and that doesn't mean they should just use their video-gaming muscles! Don't go to fast-food restaurants that don't offer you wholesome, healthy options! We the people can make a difference. We just need to change our behavior and — most important of all — our attitudes and mindset. *The MindBody FX Lifestyle* is about how you can create a new mindset that will create the changes you must make to be healthy...and it's a lot easier to be happy when healthy and to be wealthier when healthier. Why not make the decision to be healthier? If you have a strong reason—one revolving around you, not someone else—you're more likely to be successful.

Instead of giving myself reasons why I can't,
I give myself reasons why I can.

— Unknown Author

Moving Past Denial...
to Your True Self

Moving past denial is the first step toward achieving your ideal weight. For many people, denial is a constant companion — so much so that they don't realize they're world-class deniers. Don't believe me? Let's take a quick test.

Most people you meet will tell you they're "fine," no matter what you ask. How are you? Fine. How's your family? Fine. How's your job? Fine.

In reality, most of us are usually not fine at all; we can think of many aspects of our lives that we'd like to change. Perhaps we're dissatisfied with our job, co-workers or boss. Maybe our family life is either stressful, in chaos or lonely. Each person who's ever walked the planet has experienced the frustration of wanting to be more, do more and have more. Yet most of us float through life never being consciously aware of what we do or why — we tell ourselves we're fine — and that includes the way we eat. Americans spend billions of dollars each year on diet pills, books or programs that promise to transform their lives into what they dream about...believing these easy fixes will solve all their problems. Before you read any further, you need to understand that there's no magic pill to help you reach your ideal weight; *The MindBody FX Lifestyle* is based on science, and it takes commitment to achieve. And, you should already know that no amount of money, no person, no medical procedure, and no program will ever bring you total happiness; that's up to you!

You're In Control...to Stop Denying

Only you have the power to change the course of your life. You determine how you live, how you respond to life, and how much abundance you'll experience. The power to choose your life and the ability to change anything that you don't like lies totally within you.

You may be thinking, "If this is true, then why do I feel so trapped? I don't believe that I'd ever choose to be overweight." This is a completely normal reaction. The only way to understand how to improve your life is to look within. It's a challenge to understand why you think and act the way you do. By reading this book, you've chosen to undertake that challenge, and recognize who you are and how you've created your current life. Awareness is a necessity before you can change. You must understand where you are right now and how you got there; only then can you create something better.

Denial, according to Wikipedia, "is a defense mechanism in which a person is faced with a fact that is too painful to accept and rejects it instead, insisting that it is not true despite what may be overwhelming evidence. The subject may deny the reality of the unpleasant fact altogether (simple denial), admit the fact but deny its seriousness (minimization), or admit both the fact and seriousness but deny responsibility (transference). The concept of denial is particularly important to the study of addiction."

Food, like tobacco and alcohol, can become an addiction. We've all heard someone say, "I need chocolate!" or "I can't watch hockey without pizza and beer!" We all know young children who see candy in a colorful wrapper and will kick and scream until they get it. These people are addicted…and they are in denial about it.

Denial can actually be deadly. For instance, the signs of a heart attack are so varied and complex that they're often ignored and shrugged off as heartburn. I know of a young, vigorous firefighter trained in first aid and rescue who felt chest pains at the station one day. Instead of informing his colleagues, he chocked it up to the pizza he had for lunch and carried on to the end of his shift. Driving home, he finally admitted to himself that he was in so much pain that he ought to stop at the hospital. He was lucky he did; it turned out that his "indigestion" was a heart attack. He could easily have collapsed and died during a rescue or by crashing his car, leaving behind a wife and two children, all because he denied his symptoms.

We know that what we put into our bodies can eventually lead to illnesses such as diabetes, heart disease and cancer. So why do we continue to eat processed foods, trans fat and refined sugars? We're living in a state of denial. It won't happen to me. The effects of denial aren't easily measured, seen, or even felt for years, sometimes decades, but a life of excess eventually catches up to you.

Denial When It Comes to Your Weight

Here are some examples of the levels of denial—simple denial, minimization and transference—as they relate to weight.

1. **Simple Denial:** Ignoring the Facts Altogether

    These are the people who have diabetes and high blood pressure, take all kinds of medication, and continue to eat sugary cereals and chocolate bars.

2. **Minimization:** Acknowledging the Truth But Denying Its Seriousness

    These are the people who tell everyone that they've been instructed by a doctor to reduce weight, yet they continue to chow down on cheeseburgers and fries.

3. **Transference:** Acknowledging the Facts and Seriousness, But 3 Denying Responsibility

    These are the people who say, "I know I'm fat and I have diabetes, and it can kill me, but my family won't change how they eat and it's too much trouble to make separate meals for myself. I can't change."

Pay attention to your denials. Think about this. Notice what you're thinking, doing and saying. You might be saying, "I'm not in denial about anything!" — Which is a denial in itself. Your denial may be as simple as, "a piece of that pecan pie before bed won't hurt," or it could be as complex as, "sure, I'm a happy enough person." If you become aware that you deny things, people, or events in your life, don't panic. I have good news: *You have the power within you to change.*

Understanding Your True Self

When you get home at the end of the day and are alone, who are you? Your true self is who you are when no one's looking, when no one's judging, and when you can live as you please and eat what you want. Indeed, everyone has a public and private self. There's the person we show to the world, and the person who only we know…and these two selves are often very different.

When you're at work or going about your daily activities, you may consciously alter your behavior to match the person you want other people to see. For example, maybe you order a salad for lunch with co-workers, but then scarf down a burger and fries in the car on your way home. We all do this to some extent, but if your public and private food selves are quite different, this duality can be costly from a health perspective. Portraying an inauthentic version of who you are to the world can cost you in terms of stress, energy, honesty and self-worth.

You may be afraid to let others see the real you for fear of being criticized or embarrassed. The problem is that your self-image takes a hit every time you escape into denial, because what you project conflicts with your true idea of your inner self. For example, the way you dress and the things you have around you are all projections of who you believe yourself to be. A good example would be people who wear nothing but black, thinking that doing so will hide their weight. Who does this really fool? Or how about those who never eat dessert in public, but feed a sweet tooth in the privacy of their homes? The truth hurts; denial is the path of least resistance. The reality is that you and you alone have created your present current situation. No amount of covering up or denial will change that. You can't hide from who and what you really are.

The Role of Self-Worth

Our self-worth is tied very closely to our inner self. Self-worth can be described as a personal judgment of worthiness that's expressed in the attitudes we hold about ourselves, pictures that are intimately connected to our "self-value." A healthy self-worth means having a positive, constructive view of yourself and your abilities. It allows you to work toward your goals and engage in rewarding relationships. An unhealthy self-worth means having a negative, pessimistic or disapproving view of yourself, and being unable to see beyond your limitations and problems. People with an unhealthy self-worth believe they can't reach goals or have meaningful relationships...and negativity is often directly reflected in their weight and overall health. Self-destructive behavior, such as overeating or smoking, reveals a negative self-image.

You can change your self-worth, although it takes more effort than repeating a few positive phrases and receiving passing approval from others. It goes much deeper. Positive thinking and affirmations are essential, but improvement also involves taking action. ***To truly BE great, you must first think it, then believe it, and then set goals to make it happen.***

For example, let's say one day you're feeling a bit down because you've gained a few pounds...then a good friend comes along and compliments you on your appearance. This makes you feel good — temporarily. The emotion is fleeting because you know you've gained weight and have done nothing to earn or "deserve" that praise. You don't feel worthy and therefore you refuse to accept it.

Now let's assume that you've started a new workout regime and have lost four pounds in the last week. When this same friend compliments you, you feel good, and the emotion lasts. The difference is that you took action, so you feel worthy of the praise. When you take steps to improve yourself, you automatically improve the image you hold of yourself in your mind, and that affects the attitude you project. Self-worth has less to do with feeling good than it does with feeling right. Make no mistake; there's a substantial difference between the two. This feeling of right has nothing to do with right versus wrong. It's about feeling genuine and authentic inside.

You may be thinking that you haven't felt right in a very long time. You don't feel good about yourself or your overall health. You know you should skip the morning donut and coffee, but you're in a hurry and it's easy. Lunch should include vegetables or fruit, but a hot dog is quick. In fact, it may have been months since you actually had fresh, green vegetables. Your stressful life convinces you that you're doing the best you can — but are you? Each day you make small choices that together form the landscape of your life.

When you're forced to perform under stress, whether that stress is a ticking clock, traffic accident, or screaming child, your true nature shows itself very clearly. Your ingrained habits and belief systems take over, and you live on autopilot, no matter what you say you really want. Thus, denial becomes your constant companion, alleviating the guilt and burying the true causes of your unhealthy lifestyle.

Why not just go on a diet and get in shape? According to a recent dieting survey of 500 adults by Health/Insight Express, 25% of people who've tried to reduce weight have done so using at least 20 different diets. In addition, more than 60% of all dieters regained the pounds they lost...and then some, after getting tired of the routine of less food and more exercise.

This has been true for decades, but if it's really so, why do some people reduce literally hundreds of pounds and keep it off while others don't? The difference lies in the mind. Successful dieters changed their mindsets and believed they could achieve their goals. The problem with most people who struggle with their weight is that they view it as a temporary issue to be fixed rather than a lifestyle to be lived. Thus, they look for quick solutions such as harmful fad diets. They don't make the effort to establish healthy eating habits that they can maintain long term.

Few people ever take the time to develop a true plan for a healthy life. Most of the people you see each day are living on autopilot, doing exactly the same things they did the day before, learning nothing new, and experiencing the same results. They're doing time in a prison of their own making, unaware of the life they're missing.

IF YOU BELIEVE YOU CAN OR CAN'T, YOU'RE RIGHT! What are you going to decide to believe right now?

Don't Put It Off

Procrastination can be a big obstacle to attaining your ideal weight. Many people put off diet changes, saying, "I'll start tomorrow, or next Monday, or on New Year's Day." They tell themselves they're too busy to focus, and they'll get to it later. They might go so far as to commit to going to the gym and even buy a membership, but they never go.

"Put off today what you can do tomorrow" is the procrastinator's motto. Procrastination is a type of paralysis. You may look at other people being productive and feel like you have a ton of bricks on your lap and can't move. The indecision and sheer inertia of sitting still can play havoc on your plans to reach your goals.

Contrary to how it may feel sometimes, we all have the same amount of time in any given day — no more, no less. Time doesn't discriminate. Without a commitment of time, you won't change your health habits and you won't reach your goal of attaining the weight that's best for you. You'll continue to stumble through your life, accepting your behavior rather than creating what you desire.

You make a subconscious choice to procrastinate. That means you have the ability to make a conscious choice to get out of your own way. You're the cause and the effect. Become accountable for your inaction. Design a chart on which you put a gold star for every time you reach the end of your day having made good food choices and exercised, per your plan. Place a red "X" on the chart every time you slip. Set a certain number of Xs that you can't go past, say five in a month. If you have five or fewer Xs at the end of the month, then treat yourself to a special reward (not food-related!).

Another good way to get things done quickly and efficiently is to learn to say NO to people and situations that may not be important but can take you off track. For instance, perhaps you're all set to exercise when your best friend phones asking you to go to a movie instead. Many people would use the invitation as an excuse to get out of exercising. This may help your social life, but it won't help your waistline.

A great way to deal with procrastination is to use the KISS strategy: Keep it simple, silly. Let's say you're indecisive about what to eat everyday or what exercise to do. Peel off all the layers and go with the easiest solution. Walk around the block. Eat chicken and salad. You don't need to make an elaborate dinner or plan to become a gold-medal athlete overnight. You just need to do something every day to move closer to your ideal weight.

For a moment, set aside your fears of what others think, what happened in the past, and what you have to do tomorrow. Let it go and focus on this:

- What would your life be like if you reached the weight at which you are most confident?

- How would your life change?

- What would you accomplish for yourself and your family?

- What greatness would come to you, and how would your confidence and belief in yourself be affected?

Focus on these things and let go of anything holding you back.

Few people expect greatness, abundance or happiness…but you can make a choice to expect great things. You must focus on plenty, not scarcity, and on success rather than failure. Achieving a new and healthy life won't be easy at first, but it will be one of the most rewarding gifts you ever give yourself. Today is your chance to focus and look for what's rightfully yours. You deserve to have and be anything your mind can create in all areas of your life. Let's begin with achieving your ideal weight.

3 *Focusing on Your Ideal Weight*

What's the weight at which you feel most confident? There are numerous charts and measures that tell you what the suggested weight should be for your height, gender and age. Ignore all of those. Your ideal weight is about how you feel physically and emotionally. **It's whatever you want it to be.** It's about how you interact with other people, what makes you feel great in your clothes, your right dress size, how much energy you need to get through your day, whether or not your knees hurt, or whether you're healthy. You may need to shed or add pounds. You may simply want to feel healthier, or be able to walk up a flight of stairs without getting winded. You may just want to be able to zip up your pants without sucking in your stomach and not have it roll out over your waistband. Whatever it is for you — what makes you feel confident, self-assured, sexy, healthy, strong, vibrant, and free — that's your ideal weight.

Weight is not something to be cured; it's something to be managed. Individuals who've achieved their ideal weight aren't lucky or superhuman, even though they may seem that way to you. They've consciously or subconsciously made a decision to be healthy.

You may remember the old adage, "Early to bed, early to rise, makes a man healthy, wealthy, and wise." This time-honored saying can be interpreted to mean that it's your will that creates your destiny. When I hear it, I picture people who go to bed early, eat well, exercise, listen to their bodies, and are kind to themselves…and know they're rewarded with health, wealth and wisdom. They know what it takes to reach their goals. **They don't foolishly stand by and let life manage them; they manage their lives.** To be at your ideal weight, you must make the decision to do what's necessary to move you in the direction of your goal.

Always remember that your ideal weight is much more than a number. Don't become obsessed with weighing yourself every day. Don't focus on the number; that can actually be a detriment to releasing weight. Determine whether you're motivated or de-motivated by weighing yourself. If it motivates you, go ahead and weigh yourself, but limit your "scale sessions" to once a week at most. If it de-motivates you, then avoid the scale altogether and gauge your success by how you feel, the compliments you receive, the milestones you pass, the changes in your overall fitness and health, and how well your clothing fits. Good health isn't about achieving a perfect number; it's about improving your life. The changes in what you eat and the way you do things will affect your overall weight, but this isn't a race or competition. It's a lifestyle change. If you do want to chart your progress, I suggest measuring yourself monthly in a few key areas such as your chest, waist, hips, and thighs.

Modify Your Belief System

The belief you can change is the key to achieving just about anything; it encourages commitment to the process and enhances the likelihood of success. Only you can know your exact circumstances, and only you can find the solution, but if you don't believe there is a solution in the first place, you'll never find it. Stopping and searching for solutions takes time and effort. Many people are so convinced they'll fail, that they aren't willing to even try to change.

You might believe that you're so overweight that only a miracle will help you at this point, so you don't even try. No answer ever revealed itself to someone who wasn't searching. So listen up all you couch potatoes: you need to get off the couch, create a plan, stick to it, and remember that the one thing you can know for certain is that another day of watching TV will NOT help you achieve your ideal weight. No one has ever lost weight sitting in front of the TV snacking on chips and popcorn. It's time to do something. NO MORE EXCUSES!

This is not to say that change is easy. People don't change their lives with a snap of their fingers. Although your awareness of your capabilities and the perception of your current reality may change in an instant, modifying the circumstances of and relationships in your life usually takes more effort. However, these repeated efforts are critical to bringing about lasting change.

There are really only two basic reasons that people change:

1. Circumstances make them change.
2. They choose to change.

You see the truth in these two statements every day. Let's consider the first one. Have you ever gone to the doctor and been told you must reduce weight or suffer dire health consequences? Have you ever experienced a time when you needed your body to perform — maybe you were forced to walk a long distance or climb a long set of stairs — and found you just couldn't do it? Change for many people only occurs as a result of distress. If you choose to see these events for what they are, and don't attach your self-worth or emotions to them, they can be catalysts for positive change.

If a doctor warns you that you have to reduce weight or risk serious illness or even death, let that be the catalyst to a new lifestyle. If you're frightened by the fact that you couldn't climb a few flights of stairs in an emergency, let that be a lesson in about the importance of being fit. Whatever you do, don't view these events as an indicator of who you are as a person; the results can be devastating. Distressful events will happen in your life, but your reaction to those events determines the outcome. Those reactions are 100% your choice.

Now let's take a look at the second possibility — that you choose to change. How many times do you see a diet guru on TV and feel guilty that you're sitting on the couch with a bag of cookies? Or perhaps a friend or family member offered to work out with you and you found some excuse not to? Have you nagged yourself about reducing weight and promised to start next Monday? Does all that guilt and nagging mean that you'll change? No. You'll only change the way you do things by choice — when you truly want to change and are ready to do so. You'll never be nagged, pressured or pushed by someone else into lasting change.

You must decide that you want to change. Not next week or next year — RIGHT NOW! Urgency is a key component to making serious and lasting changes, and the decision to change is necessary. Why? Because you're more likely to act on — and stick to — your own decisions rather than someone else's. You must decide for yourself that you want to change, not because your children, spouse or parents say you should. Not because your doctor or fitness coach says it's the right thing to do. Not because some "expert" says so. You must decide to change to a healthy lifestyle because you want to and because you've made the choice to do so.

The Power Of You

Human beings always act and feel and perform in accordance with what they imagine to be true about themselves and their environment.
— Dr. Maxwell Maltz

The idea that we create our own reality is downright painful for many, or at least distasteful. Many people honestly believe they have no choices, and even those who do believe they can choose often beat themselves up for past choices they've made — diet failures, lack of fitness — the results of which they're living right now.

We're totally responsible for whatever manifests in our lives — all of it. This again begs the question, why would we create bodies that are overweight, fatigued, stressed out and not physically fit? Why would we choose to do any of that to ourselves? No one creates these things deliberately, yet we've all done it at one time or another. The key to changing is to understand exactly HOW we do it. What is the process of creation, of manifestation?

Many people have heard of the Law of Attraction, which basically states that you get what you focus on. Unfortunately, many people who think they're focusing on creating their ideal weight are really focusing on pounds. For example, have you ever set a goal, perhaps even written it down, to achieve a certain clothing size? Did you then spend your days constantly hopping on the scale? Worrying over each pound? Continually calculating how many pounds had to disappear and in what time frame? While your goal was to achieve a certain clothing size, you spent most of your time focusing on pounds and that, therefore, is what you attracted.

The reverse is also true. When you focus on what you want, whether it's a certain clothing size or your ideal weight, you'll manifest only that. For instance, let's say you want to be a size 8. Focus on the clothing size and imagine yourself wearing size 8 — how it feels to put on size 8 clothes, eating as a person who already wears a size 8 — then your mind will focus on becoming a size 8. The same holds true for your ideal weight. Perhaps your dream is to weigh 140 pounds. The key is not to concentrate on how many fewer pounds you need to weigh to successfully attain that goal; the key is to imagine yourself as already weighing 140 pounds, thinking as you would if you were 140 pounds, exercising like a person who weighs 140 pounds, and making the food choices a 140-pound person makes. **See it, believe it, feel it, and be it. It's a simple concept, but quite foreign for most people.**

As we mature, we have experiences that shape who we are and what we believe. These experiences may be good or bad, but each event causes us to make a decision about what we believe, and that decision, in turn, affects how we live our lives from that point forward. The belief systems or programs set in place at a very young age affect and alter the way we see the world. For example, if you were constantly told to clean your plate, that habit may carry into adulthood. If you were encouraged and praised for good grades rather than for playing sports, you may have decided that intelligence is more important than being physically fit. If you were hurt in a relationship or lonely as a child, you may have decided that you can't trust other people and found that additional weight is a way to keep them away. These belief systems and programs that were set in place when you were a child persist through your life. They affect your attitudes and feelings toward food and overall health, and manifest in your life through actions and behaviors that produce your personal outcomes.

You can see how events we experience as children are carried forward as beliefs into adulthood. It's been said that about 80% of what children believe about themselves is in place by the time they're 4 years old. From the ages of 4 to 8, another 10% of children's beliefs are constructed. By the age of 18, 95% of what we believe about ourselves has been formed and produces the perspective from which we view and make sense of our world. As we've all had different experiences, we each see the world slightly differently. This means we don't necessarily see things as they are; we perceive them through the filter of our beliefs. Thus, we create our own version of reality.

Effecting Change

Human beings have the ability to ponder the past and use its lessons to change the future. However, few people stop to evaluate what they believe about themselves or why. Belief systems and habits learned from events, family or your environment can move you forward or hold you back from successfully transforming your life. One of the first steps to change is to ask why.

Years ago, I heard a story about a woman who was baking a ham. Her daughter asked why she cut the ends off it prior to baking, expecting to hear some great culinary secret. Her reply was, "Because that's the way my grandmother did it." The young girl went to her grandmother and asked the same question. Her grandmother replied, "Because that's the way my mother did it." The young girl then went to her great-grandmother, who was quite old and fragile, and asked her why she cut the ends off the ham. The old woman replied, "Because we were very poor and didn't have a baking pan large enough unless I cut the ends off."

This is a simple illustration of adopting someone else's belief systems without knowing all the facts. Old rules don't necessarily make sense in new environments or circumstances, yet they continue to be passed on. This is especially noticeable in people's beliefs about food. Why do you think people who are overweight all their lives tend to produce children who are also overweight? Or, why do you think that wealthy people often raise children who continue to attract wealth? Are these groups of people that different? Absolutely not; in fact, in most ways they're the same. One big difference, however, is their mindset.

Overweight people tend to focus on their inability to reduce weight, thus attracting more weight and creating a belief that they're overweight. In other words, they think of themselves as fat, and therefore they become so. Wealthy people focus on wealth, so it seems they attain it more easily. They think wealthy. With this positive attraction type of thinking, many people who were born to poverty have become wealthy. Think of the Oprah's of the world — they used the power of their minds to move from being poor to becoming some of the wealthiest people on the planet.

It isn't luck that changes such people's lives for the better; it's will and determination, and the thoughts they think. It's knowing they can achieve whatever they set out to accomplish. People who are struggling financially often say they are broke. By thinking this, by accepting this circumstance, they will stay broke. If they changed their thinking to, "I am financially secure," they would much more easily become just that. You can trick your mind into thinking whatever it is you want to think; you just have to be aware of your thoughts and their context.

Just as poverty can be a state of mind, so can obesity. Everyone who's overweight can choose to succeed at becoming fit and healthy, but it must be a conscious and sincere choice...beginning with a decision to have a healthy and abundant mindset. Even if you can't immediately change where you live, work, or play, you can immediately change your perspective of the world. By doing this, you create the desire and passion necessary to aggressively pursue the healthy life you deserve.

To receive a Free Special Report called Tips and Tools for Implementing a Healthier Lifestyle go to **www.mindbodyfx.com/specialreport1**.

Watch your thoughts; they become words.
Watch your words; they become actions.
Watch your actions; they become habits.
Watch your habits; they become character.
Watch your character; it becomes your destiny.

— Frank Outlaw

4   *Creating a New Mindset*

You are today where your thoughts have brought you.
You will be tomorrow where your thoughts take you.

— James Allen

We've all heard the phrase, "You are what you eat." I'd like to add to that: you are what you think. What you eat is the manifestation of what you think. As discussed in the previous chapters, to understand how to change your thinking about achieving your ideal weight, you must first understand how your mind works.

The mind is an incredibly powerful tool, yet few of us ever stop to think about what creates our thought patterns, feelings and actions. Therefore, we have no idea what's responsible for how we experience our lives. The answer lies in the concept of attitude.

When we think of attitude, most people envision a type of positive thinking or having a bright and cheery demeanor. While that's an important aspect of attitude, it's just one component. Attitude is a composite of your thoughts, feelings, and actions — not one of the three, but all of them working together in seamless combination. These thoughts, feelings, and actions are a product of your conditioned behavior, which includes how you were raised, how you've been educated, and who's influenced our lives. You're the product of your individual experiences, so you have a unique attitude concerning your health and fitness. To understand how these ideas and actions become ingrained in your behavior, it helps to understand how you learn.

Beginning right now, you'll learn how to take responsibility, live in the present and not the past, work through your fears, and stop denying and procrastinating. Everything you know you've learned in four stages:

1. **Unconscious Incompetence**

2. **Conscious Incompetence**

3. **Conscious Competence**

4. **Unconscious Competence**

Think about how babies learn to walk. They first crawl to move around, not knowing any other way and maybe not even knowing that there is any other way (unconscious incompetence). Eventually, babies recognize there's another way to move, and soon develop the desire to walk, yet they still haven't mastered the technique and have to settle for holding onto furniture and practicing (conscious incompetence). Soon, babies learn to concentrate and take a few short steps at a time without falling (conscious competence). Finally, they become so competent that they can walk without even having to think about it; it's become second nature (unconscious competence).

Once a process is learned, you become unconsciously competent at it, so you no longer need to think about how to do it. This same process is at work when you learn to ride a bicycle, drive a car or use a computer. Let's look at this process as it relates to weight:

1. **Unconscious Incompetence** – This can also be described as what you don't know, you don't know. With respect to weight, this may be reflected in two ways: you may not even realize you have a weight problem or you may not know that you haven't had the right diet and tools to reach your ideal weight.

2. **Conscious Incompetence** – In other words, what you know you don't know. You know you have a weight problem, but you don't know what to do about it; you realize something's missing in the quest to reach your ideal weight, but what it is eludes you.

3. **Conscious Competence** – What you know, you know. You know you have a weight problem and you've even taken steps you believe will lead you to your ideal weight, but you haven't been successful in attaining it.

4. **Unconscious Competence** – What you don't know, you know. You know you have a weight problem, but you understand what you need to do to attain your ideal weight and you do it without thinking. You've harnessed the power to manage your weight by retraining your mind. This is where I want to take you with *The MindBody FX Lifestyle.*

Your mind always thinks in pictures. If I told you to think of your car, your home or your refrigerator, instantly you'd have an image of these things in your mind. This is why you're able to drive to places you've been to before, yet you often can't provide street names or house numbers, or when getting directions, you respond to landmarks instead of streets. If someone tells you to turn left at the gas station, you see it in your mind and automatically know where it is.

If I ask you to think of your mind, no picture comes to light. You might get a picture of your brain, but your brain is not your mind any more than your elbow is. Your mind exists in every cell of your body. Understanding your mind and how it works can be a difficult and abstract concept, so here's an illustration to help explain. I've used the stick person example developed in the 1930s by Dr. Thurman Fleet in San Antonio, Texas.

Conscious Mind

The top circle represents your mind or your thoughts, and the bottom circle represents your body or your actions. The mind is divided into the conscious and subconscious. The conscious mind is the area that receives all the input and experiences from the outside world. As you're faced with new events and ideas, your conscious mind has the ability to accept or reject any information it receives. When thoughts come to you from your surroundings, the conscious mind is the filter that allows you to choose only those ideas and events with which you want to be emotionally involved. The conscious mind is also where you create the dreams and goals you want for your life.

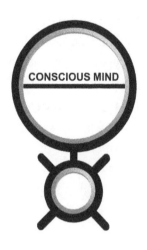

CONSCIOUS MIND

It's estimated that given today's media bombardment, you're exposed to tens of thousands of images per day. You can effectively capture or process approximately 1,000 of these images on a conscious level. The information age has increased the complexity of what you're exposed to during your life. Although in many ways this makes your life more efficient and easy, it also means that your mind must constantly choose what to process. Like most people, you probably don't think of this as an active choice, but it is. Consider two different people's accounts of the same event; how is it that they can differ so greatly when they saw and heard the same things? The discrepancy results from two brains choosing to process different images. The ones you choose will create the story you perceive as reality.

If you're constantly inundated with negative messages, you're bound to choose negative thoughts and ideas that will be stored in your subconscious mind. You then become a negative person with negative ideas and opinions — not only of the events in your life, but also of yourself. If you want to think, feel, and act more positively, you must guard your subconscious with your conscious mind by carefully choosing what ideas engage your emotions and what images you view repeatedly.

Subconscious Mind

The subconscious mind is the "emotional mind" or "feeling mind." It has only one answer to all commands it receives from the conscious mind, and that answer is "YES!"

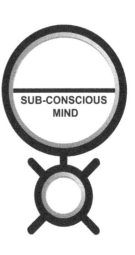

The subconscious mind has no ability to accept or reject thoughts. It's therefore important to monitor thoughts and ideas as you receive them in your conscious mind. The subconscious mind is a blank screen, and any thoughts you accept will resurface on it. If you worry about something happening, then the subconscious mind will move you in the direction of having that negative thing will happen. If you say or think you're clumsy, this thought may make you trip on a crack in the sidewalk.

Likewise, if you create positive ideas of how you want events to unfold or how you want to respond to the unfortunate things that happen in your life, then your subconscious mind can, and will, exhibit those positive results. Worrying and focusing on what you don't want takes just as much energy and time, if not more, than focusing on what you do want. You'll always attract more of the same energy with which you're in harmony, and if it's negative, then that's what you'll receive.

The encouraging message from this is that you can monitor your conscious mind. More importantly, you can teach yourself to increase your positive results, as Napoleon Hill describes in *Think and Grow Rich*. Hill encourages you to create the thoughts and ideas you want. By repeating those thoughts, you can manifest the realities in your life.

The Body

Your body is the physical form and machine that's instructed daily by your dominant thoughts and actions. It carries out actions based on directions from the conscious and subconscious mind, so it's the evidence of what's held there. For example, let's say you decide you want to be a public speaker. If you're nervous and worry about saying something inappropriate, or are concerned that someone will make fun of you, those thoughts will manifest in the body as sweaty palms, embarrassment, and stumbling over words. However, if you spend time imagining how positively your audience will respond, how articulate you'll sound, and how energized you'll feel, that will manifest

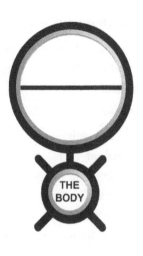

in the body as well. You'll be confident and filled with energy, and your audience can't help but respond positively. When you intentionally change the thoughts to which you give the most focus and energy, and repeat these thoughts until they become desires, they're impressed upon your subconscious mind and become emotions. Your body puts those emotions into action and your actions become your results.

The Cycle of Creating Your Results

Now that you understand how your mind works, let's discuss further how to get the results you seek. It's important to realize that no achievement started at the results stage, but began as a vision, an imagined goal. In that same vein, your journey toward achieving your ideal weight—and maintaining it—will take you through what's known as The Cycle of Creating Your Results:

- **Thoughts.** What you think is affected by how you see the world, and this defines your philosophy.

- **Feelings.** Your thoughts will lead to your feelings, which represent your attitude toward everything that happens around you.

- **Actions.** The way you act stems from the feelings you've developed based on your thoughts.

- **Results.** The cycle of thoughts leading to feelings leading to actions will produce your results. This is why you truly are in control of everything that happens to you.

- **Lifestyle.** All of your results bundled together make up your lifestyle. Again, the choices you make are going to determine the type of life you have, including how healthy you are and whether you're at your ideal weight.

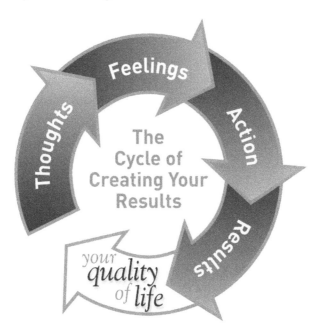

You can't choose to begin this cycle at anywhere but the beginning. This is why I continue to dwell on the importance of mindset as it relates to releasing weight. Unfortunately, there are some obstacles to changing your thought pattern, which has been ingrained since you were a child… but if you set your mind to it, you can make significant changes to your own philosophy.

As you grow older, you tend to become more rigid in your thoughts, because they've been developed based on the sum of your life experiences. When you were a child, your imagination ran wild; you thought anything was possible. That sense of suspending reality ekes out as you develop a better understanding of the world around you, but you also often lose the ability to use your imagination to its full potential.

Exercising your imagination to broaden your possibilities is an important step to take as you set any goal. Releasing weight is certainly not rocket science, but think about those scientists whose goal was to journey through the universe to land a man on the moon. Would they ever have attained their mission if they hadn't imagined that their goal was possible?

Visualization can be an important part of realizing a goal. You've already heard me say this, but you must visualize that you're at your ideal weight…imagining how it feels and how other people respond to the "new" you. Your mindset must be programmed for success, not stuck on past failures or the litany of excuses you can come up with for failing to attain your ideal weight. Keeping a personal journal can be an important part of your evolution; in addition to documenting your thoughts in real time, it can also help you think more objectively about yourself, and understand more clearly how your philosophy has been formed. I'll address journaling later in this book.

There's no getting past the fact that you may be in the Thoughts part of the creation cycle for quite some time. You simply can't flip a switch and change the way you've been thinking for your entire life. The good news is that once you've identified potential obstacles, done a serious self-inquiry regarding your commitment to follow through and quieted your mind so you're able to visualize where you want to be…you're in a great place to turn your new mindset into new feelings and actions that lead to the results you desire. You have the power to make the changes that are necessary to lead a healthy lifestyle, which goes hand in hand with attaining your ideal weight.

It may seem at first that to shift your attitude to one that promotes making decisions that support your weight-releasing goal should be simple, but as I've said before, and will say again, the fact that so many people are overweight speaks to how very difficult it is to change an ingrained attitude or belief.

While you can't change your past, you can change the way you let it affect your attitude moving forward. You must also grab control of your present; realize that you need to embrace the opportunities presented to you right now to realize the future you want to have.

The Feelings part of the cycle is where it's important to pump up your self-worth. You're a unique personality with qualities that make you different and special; if you don't believe that, why should anyone else? You must know who you are and develop an attitude that you deserve to live a healthy life…so you're ready to take the steps that will lead you there.

One difficult thing that needs to happen at this stage is taking a look at those around you, including family, friends and business colleagues, and making decisions about whether it's valuable for you to continue to associate with them. Having a support system will help you immeasurably on your journey to your ideal weight, and you really don't want to be surrounded by negativity. There will be some people you can't cut from your life—like your family—but you can explain to them how important it is to you to have their encouragement during this evolutionary process toward fulfilling your lifestyle dream.

Once you reach the Action stage, you'll have already come so far. Your thoughts and feelings will have evolved to the point where now it's time to go for it! This can actually paralyze some people, but you need to push through and begin taking steps to reach your goal. Remember that this is a process, and things can be done incrementally; "Rome wasn't built in a day."

It's important to have a plan and be disciplined at following it. Set goals that are attainable for you, realistic and not "pie-in-the-sky." The combination of planning, using your imagination and then acting accordingly can dramatically change the quality of your life…and the power is within you to do just that.

The Results stage is one that you want to aspire to remain in forever… but you shouldn't despair if you need to revisit any of the earlier steps to reinvigorate yourself. Certainly attaining, and then maintaining, your ideal weight is the gold standard result, but there are many incremental results you can track as well, rewarding yourself (without food!) for your successes.

Here are just a few results that are worth celebrating:

- Dropping one size, even if it's from 18 to 16…and you have a ways to go to reach your ideal weight
- Cutting fast food out of your diet for a week, a month or longer
- Staying away from soda for a week, a month or longer
- Keeping on track with your exercise plan, for a week, a month or longer

Even though your ultimate goal hasn't yet been reached, you're visualizing that you're already at your ideal weight…and rewarding yourself for the achievements you're having along the way. Your confidence, positive attitude and aim for maximum results will spur you forward.

When you lead a healthy lifestyle, that's a reflection of who you are, but it shouldn't be confused with a condition to be pursued. We've all heard the phrase, money doesn't buy you happiness, and indeed, we all probably know people who have many material comforts, but aren't happy.

Your lifestyle is a series of "mores": living more fully, consciously, joyfully and appreciatively. It's not a reward for making an effort, but a way to see that effort be more rewarding, meaningful and productive. As you work toward attaining your healthy lifestyle, you still need to be happy with where you are, even as you push forward to make positive, life-long changes that become subconscious habits.

For a Free Checklist to keep you on track with your goal of achieving your ideal weight go to **www.mindbodyfx.com/checklist**.

 **5** ***Taking Control of Your Habits***

I know you're already aware of what you have to do to be at your ideal weight; the problem is that you're not doing it. The secret to success is to gain an understanding of why you're not doing it, determining the primary cause of the problem and correcting it.

Paradigms

A paradigm, which can be a habit, pattern, belief, attitude, work practice or expectation, gives you the understanding to interpret and approach the world around you. When you examine your paradigms around weight, you may find that your current results are not the ones you want. Moving your conditioned results in line with what you want will support your objective of reaching your ideal weight. For instance, let's say you used to drink one glass of red wine every evening, but to reach your ideal weight you've changed that to a glass of water with a lemon slice instead. This is a paradigm shift.

We do things we know we shouldn't do — things we don't want to do — and we do them anyway. We're conditioned to believe that it's our behavior that's causing the unwanted results in our life...but that's not true. We're forever attempting to change those behavior patterns — eat less, eliminate junk foods, and exercise more often — all without success. Or, we're successful for a short period of time, but then we start going down the same street, falling into the same hole. Unfortunately, some people stay on that street for their entire life.

Trying to create a paradigm shift by changing your behavior will never work. You must first address the primary cause of the problem, which starts with your thoughts and beliefs.

There are millions of people in every country in the world going on special diets to reduce weight. These people aren't trying to reach their ideal weight; their obsession is with losing weight. There's a dual problem with this. First, they believe that food — eating the wrong food or eating too much food — is the cause of their problem, which isn't entirely true. Their eating habits are the secondary cause of their problem; the primary cause, their beliefs, must be corrected if the results are going to permanently change. Second, when you lose anything — it doesn't matter what it is, from your car keys to those 20 pounds — you're subconsciously programmed to immediately begin to looking for it. And, unfortunately, when it comes to weight loss, you usually find it.

The MindBody FX Lifestyle is designed to do what Portia Nelson described in the little poem at the beginning of the book: take you down another street.

The simplest and most comprehensive definition of a paradigm that I've ever come across is that it's a multitude of habits…concepts expressed in action without any conscious thought.

> *To ignore the power of paradigms to influence your judgmentis*
> *to put yourself at significant risk when exploring the future.*

> *To be able to shape your future you have to be ready*
> *and able to change your paradigm.*

> **— Joel Barker**

Armed with paradigms, you approach and react to the world around you, interpreting what you see and experience according to your shared understanding and certain culturally determined guidelines. A paradigm, in a sense, tells you there's a game, what it is, and how to play it successfully. A paradigm shift is changing to a new game or a new set of rules…and when the rules change, the whole world will appear to change. You're then going to go down a different street.

Our Habits

One way to change negative habits is by changing the negative beliefs you hold about yourself. Do you have a habit that confirms a belief about yourself? Is that habit serving you well, or is it confirming a "self-belief" that you wish was different? For example, do you always "super-size" your meals? If so, this is confirming a belief that you're super-sized. You may reject the idea that this is so, but actions speak louder than words. Only by choosing and committing to a new habit will you eventually change your belief about yourself, creating new proof based on your actions.

How do you begin to change your beliefs and form new, more positive and healthy habits? The first thing to do is stop lying to yourself. We all do it. How many times have you promised yourself to stick to a healthy portion size and not eat too much, and have instead gone to the fridge and eaten everything in sight?

Here's a story one of my clients told me that's a good example of what can happen when you lie to yourself:

"My girlfriend and I made a pact to get in shape last summer. We were supposed to eat healthy lunches then meet at the gym three days a week. She did great and had a wonderful positive attitude — but I didn't. I found myself hiding the fast food wrappers and making excuses for why my weight didn't change. I cringed just thinking about the gym, and more often than not, found some excuse not to go.

It wasn't long before she achieved her goal, and I constantly belittled her achievement because I felt so angry with myself for sneaking around and doing things we'd agreed not to do. The truth is, she wanted to change and I didn't. One night, when we were supposed to have dinner with her family, she called and asked me not to go. She pointed out how I'd been acting and said she wouldn't be treated that way in front of her family. I was shocked. I didn't even realize that my insecurity and anger had caused her such pain.

Three weeks and four-dozen roses later, we were at the gym every day, and I now tell everyone how proud I am of what she's accomplished. I finally made the decision to get healthy for myself, not because she wanted me to, but because I wanted to...and that made all the difference."

Small Steps

Changing your entire lifestyle may seem a little overwhelming at first, but you can ease into it by taking a few small steps to form new healthy habits.

1. **Envision the end result.** You're not changing a habit for the sake of change itself, but because doing so will get you closer to achieving or having your ideal weight. If you have a habit of watching TV for a few hours every night and munching on a bag of potato chips, then turn the TV off and substitute reading or a walk.

2. **Take a reality assessment.** What's working well, what needs improvement, and what's getting in the way of your progress? Your exercise routine of lifting weights may be going perfectly well, but what if you'd really like to find a more interesting way to tone your muscles? Put that on a list of things that are important to you and start working to make it happen.

3. **Pick a challenge – any challenge.** You don't have to pick a big challenge to start. Think in terms of improving one percent a day – something very attainable. For example, if you drink several cups of coffee or tea a day but want to get off caffeine, start by drinking one less cup per day or even one half cup less. Within a short time, you'll have weaned yourself from the habit.

4. **Action is the key.** Form a plan for staying on track. Keep a written record of your progress. It's easy to forget the little victories, but going back and looking at a journal of success – even in the smallest areas – gives you a mental boost and encourages you to stick with your plan.

By using these small steps — if you really commit to and persist with your new habits — I guarantee you'll have a new perspective and belief about who you are and what you can accomplish. Then you can move on to choosing the next healthy habit you want to develop and strengthen.

Making a Decision to Change

You develop your beliefs about what you can or can't accomplish from even the smallest events. Words spoken by a spouse, parent or friend can affect your belief in your ability to change. Although family can be supportive, they also remember every failure and often point them all out. You may have family or friends who constantly tell you that you're fine the way you are and just to accept it…but if you don't feel fine, then you're not. You have to decide if you'll let other people limit your life.

You must remember that it's not what you're born with or without that determines who you'll become. By the same token, you can't blame others for your success or failure, as this is the road to irresponsibility and helplessness. You can only change yourself and the way you interact with others. This is the path to true happiness and success.

Knowing that you're in complete and total control of your own destiny, no matter what happens or what others say is very empowering and gives you the freedom to create the life that you desire and become the person you really want to be.

A significant roadblock to change can be the "poor me" syndrome or victim mentality, which is stifling; you can get caught, feeling powerless in your ability to move forward. Do you constantly cry about your lot in life — I'm too fat! I have no friends! — yet still sit at home alone on the couch in front of the TV rather than doing something about it, like joining a hiking club where you can meet other people and get some exercise at the same time? You certainly know people who are like this. Have you ever been to dinner at a family member's house and "Cousin Sally" is sitting sulking in a chair, not participating in the conversation because she's having a bad day? Do you know someone who's constantly blaming the cat, the car, or his boss for whatever went wrong that day? We all do it occasionally — fall into the trap of playing the victim and the blame game. No more! You need to be done with that if you truly want to achieve your dreams!

Once you become aware of the victim mentality, you'll discover immediately how negative and destructive it really is. You'll also find that you're not really a victim, in most circumstances, except in your own mind. You have the power to change if you want to. Many people, unfortunately, move from a victim mentality to an excuse mentality. By choosing to shift blame to something other than themselves, they don't take ownership of their own lives or health. You frequently see this if you ask people why they've given up their exercise routines or resumed bad habits. They'll offer excuses rather than acknowledge that they chose to take that action — no one made them. Many people never realize that they've excused themselves right out of living and have started down a destructive path that leads to death. Alcoholics Anonymous has a saying: "There are a million excuses for picking up a drink, but no good reason." Excuses abound for not living a healthy life, but real reasons are few. Stop making excuses and choose to change for the better.

To break the vicious cycle of excuses, half-truths, and anger with which you've been living, you must first make a decision. By mastering the art of decision-making, you'll bring more benefit to your life than any other lesson you could learn.

Decision makers are the movers and shakers of the world. They're leaders, and because of that, they become successful. How do they do that? They understand that every decision is actually the answer to a question. Every action has an equal and opposite reaction: up – down; right – wrong; inside – outside; yes – no; cold – hot; black – white; question – answer; fat – thin. The laws of the universe hold the answer to any question; you just need to know how to tune into that frequency.

By understanding this and altering your life as a result, you'll find that you're able to make good decisions and reach your potential — in this case, achieving the weight you desire. Making a decision brings order to your existence, and order brings results. Let's say you make the decision to reach your ideal weight. By deciding to lay out the framework of the plan, you set yourself up for success. Simply moving forward without a plan will bring failure. This is indecision. That in itself is a decision you make — but not the right one, not the one that will work with the laws of the universe and attract what you want.

Indecision and lack of planning create all-out mental wars and emotional turmoil or ambivalence. The result is having both positive and negative feelings toward something or someone, so you're pulled in opposite directions: leave – don't leave; do it – don't do it; go – don't go; say it – don't say it; drink it – don't drink it; eat it – don't eat it. Eliminate these wars within yourself and you can become an effective decision maker. This takes courage; you must have the courage to believe you can make the right decision.

What If?

The most difficult step for many of us is conquering a debilitating mindset of "can't." We allow our pre-established beliefs about our own limitations to blot out any productive thought process that might lead to self-improvement.

Whether by virtue of your inner self-vision, or the chains that others (or society as a whole) have placed on you, you may have become totally unable to contemplate a successful result. As long as this remains the case, ultimate success is unlikely (if not impossible). Unlocking the powerful potential of vision and desire will create the momentum to take you to your goal. That won't be achieved as long as the paralyzing mental block, the debilitating "can't" outlook, remains in your path.

Conquering this mental block can start with two simple (but powerful) words: what if? My attorney (of all people!) believes that these are the two most powerful words in our language. They are the keys to lifting a dark shroud of defeat and allowing in a beam of positive, progressive light.

His view is that every grand human achievement, every startling accomplishment — which to that point had seemed inconceivable — started with the words: what if? What if humans could achieve flight? What if it was possible to transmit sound and pictures along wires? What if diseases like polio could be defeated? What if people could travel to the moon and the stars (and back!)? What if a woman could become prime minister of England and an African American could become the U.S. president?

Every one of these accomplishments was achieved because someone was willing to contemplate the possible rather than be limited by the impossible. These people evaded the paralytic burden of a prior inability to achieve – or even imagine – that result. Having done so, it was (simply put) just a matter of thinking about how the result might someday be achieved.

To someone who focuses on the possible, the question, "What if humans could achieve flight?" soon leads to asking, "What would the result look like? What would have to be accomplished along the way to make it happen? What challenges would I have to overcome? Where's the best place to start?" You can think like this, too; once you begin allowing your mind to contemplate possibilities, the future can become a wide-open landscape.

Robert Smithson is a labor and employment attorney based in Kelowna, BC. He has no particular background in the context of weight management or psychology or coaching. What he *does* do is deal every day with people who have, for one reason or another, lost their jobs. He has first-hand knowledge that the loss of a job is one of the two or three most stressful events we experience. Its impact goes to the heart of who we think we are and it quickly undermines our hard-won feelings of self-confidence and self-worth.

The immediate challenge faced by many people who've just lost their jobs is that they simply cannot envision the possibility that this event may prove to be the best thing that ever happened to them. They can't, or won't, imagine that this will be the beginning of a whole new, exciting phase of their life. They can't entertain the thought that this may be a milestone they'll someday look back on as having kick-started them to seek out the career they've always wanted. They're paralyzed by what's just happened.

It's important to understand that not everyone receives the news of a job loss in the same manner. Robert tells of having represented people who, in their minds, have already moved on to the next phase of their work life before the details of their departure from their former job have been wrapped up. This book isn't aimed at those people. It's for the people who, for whatever reason, would allow the loss of a job to hang on them like an anchor; these people will benefit from a "what if?" dose.

Robert is challenged when dealing with those who react poorly to changing circumstances. Their negative outlook creates an additional burden for him. They often have difficulty making decisions, they can be unresponsive to requests for input and information, and their pessimism clouds their ability to recognize a positive result.

In Robert's view, these folks need to allow themselves the luxury, even briefly, of setting aside their mental block and focusing on "what if?" scenarios. What if there's another employer out there looking for someone just like me? What if this time away from the rush of daily work is what I need to gather my thoughts and rediscover who I am? What if there's another workplace out there that's the perfect fit for the type of person I am? What if I made use of this opportunity to train for the career I've always wanted? What if I've been chasing a career that I never really wanted to begin with?

The beauty of this simple thought process is that it frees you to imagine the possible. It opens up the horizon of potential in a way that, stuck behind the debilitating mindset of "can't," you'd never have accessed. By distracting your mind from the mental block, from the impossible, it allows a progressive, healing thought process to commence. It's sort of a comfortable first step, or a halfway point, between "can't" and "can."

Once the "what if?" process has begun, it can create a momentum of its own and can shrink (or even eliminate) the mental block. It can generate excitement, anticipation, and an eagerness you previously thought impossible. Your "can't" outlook shifts into "can" mode, and suddenly the mental block is behind you. What lies ahead is a world full of previously inconceivable possibilities.

What this achieves for Robert's purposes are clients who've regained their focus, can make rational decisions, and are open to strategies that will lead to a positive resolution. Can this thought process work in the context of changing your way of thinking about achieving your ideal weight? I know it can.

The biggest "what if" question for you right now is: what if it *is* possible for me to achieve my ideal body weight?

The choices you make, make you.

— **John C Maxwell**

6 ## *Becoming Your Vision*

Rule your mind or it will rule you.

— Horace

If you're like many people, you've tried numerous diets and perhaps even had some success, but have slowly returned to your old weight and habits because of your old beliefs. Why does this happen? It almost seems as if your body conspires against you at times, but the true culprit is your mindset. There's a weight that you're comfortable with (your comfort zone). You wear it like an old sweater. It makes you feel safe and secure. You don't even know you're enabling the beliefs and habits that keep it on, but you are.

People naturally resist ambiguity and uncertainty. Contemplating weight reduction is no exception. When you don't know what's to come, you get fearful and lose the ability or desire to move forward; it's human nature to stay in your comfort zone. Ironically, you keep yourself from succeeding, and then are confused when you don't.

No matter what area of your life you want to change, you'll experience this same phenomenon, whether it's weight, relationships or career. You live your life mostly on autopilot, following the deep-rooted habits you've created over time. You don't even consciously think about these beliefs and habits until someone else points them out. This is often the case when people are asked how much they eat in a day. They'll usually say a very normal or even small amount. However, if their eating habits were monitored, you'd find they often actually eat two to three times the amount they say they do. They aren't lying. They simply eat so much out of habit that they really don't remember everything that goes into their mouths.

It may seem to be a very simple task to change these beliefs and habits and create new ones, but it takes more effort than you might think. By their very definition, beliefs and habits are entrenched in your subconscious, and it takes extensive repetition to replace one belief or habit with another. This is the time when it seems your body is fighting your efforts, but it's not your body at all, only your subconscious programming. How many times have you started a diet, lost 10 or maybe even 20 pounds, then watched those pounds creep right back — and maybe bring along a few friends? This is your subconscious mind at work. Even if the range of weight that you've become accustomed to is morbidly obese, your mind has accepted this as where you want to be—because that's you. It's your comfort zone. Therefore, while you may achieve success at the beginning of a weight reduction program, you lose interest or the ability to move forward.

When the change you want to implement starts to move you out of your comfort zone, you have feelings of uncertainty and apprehension. People respond to you differently and you act differently. Fear of this unknown territory, even if the change is positive, can inhibit your ability to continue because it goes against what you've come to accept as your self-image. If you believe yourself to be unattractive, then reduce your weight and start getting compliments, that's good, right? Yes and no. Of course, it's great to get positive feedback, but it also puts you in the position of gaining more attention from others, which could make you uncomfortable, as you may feel your efforts are being scrutinized. Before you know it, you regain all your weight in a subconscious effort to relieve the stress of being noticed.

The only way to change this behavior is to know that the change will happen and accept it as so. When you really and truly know something will happen, there's no trace of doubt, no lingering thread of skepticism. A great analogy when referring to how this knowing works is called the XY Factor.

The X Factor is the conditioning that resonates in the subconscious mind. You can think of it as a habit. A good example of this might be a woman who wants to reduce her weight by 20 pounds. She's heard of the latest diets and has attempted weight reduction over the years. She thinks she knows what works for her and what doesn't. She may have learned poor eating habits from her mother and now passes her beliefs about food onto her family. This is her comfort zone.

The Y Factor can be anything that represents change. It disrupts what we you know and makes you uncomfortable. Now let's assume this same woman sets a target of achieving her ideal weight by summer. She wants to reach that target. Achieving it could change her life in great ways. It's very important to her.

It's when the conscious mind makes the decision to accept Y that the X Factor feels threatened. Everything this woman has known and experienced rebels against this new idea and right away fear sets in. When fear enters the picture, logic leaves. Concentrating on that fear attracts more of the same and the goal seems even further away. This is the point where many people may give up. Doubts become overwhelming, and the subconscious begs to retreat back into what it's known — back into the comfort zone.

You can fight back. Tackle your fears; only you can let them win. You know now that by concentrating on the positive goal ahead and setting those fears aside, you're imprinting new ideas into your subconscious. If you do this enough and concentrate on the changes you want to make and the goals you're trying to achieve, you're allowing Y to win. You're empowering your mind with new thoughts, resulting in different actions that produce the results you desire.

Imagery/Visualization and the Law of Attraction

You often have difficulty thinking in abstract ideas; you even dream in full-color movie clips! Imagery, also called visualization, is a process you use, even if you don't know you're doing it; it's just how you naturally think. If you think about reducing your weight, you don't conjure up fat cells shriveling or healthy foods being digested better by your body. You imagine how it would look and feel to be at your ideal weight — what new clothes you might wear or what kind of compliments you might receive.

It's important to understand how imagery and the Law of Attraction work in harmony. The Law of Attraction states that you will attract more of whatever you focus on. This can be alarming because whatever you're thinking about repeatedly, whatever you're mulling over or grumbling about, even if only to yourself, that's imagery — which invokes the Law of Attraction. This phenomenon starts in your thinking mind (conscious mind), is amplified by your emotional mind (subconscious mind), and manifests in your body (through actions).

Your body, like all matter, is made up entirely of energy, so you send out vibrations or energy. This energy attracts more of the same, so whatever you've been imagining, good or bad, is reflected back to you. You have the ability to choose what you want to focus on or imagine, and as a result, the vibrations you send out. Even if the goal or result you desire seems outrageous, your subconscious mind doesn't know the difference between the real and imagined circumstances. Many people report that significant achievements can be reached after just 30 days of imagining a goal, circumstance or material object. This is not to say that any goal can be completely accomplished in a single month, only that you'll be well on the path to achieving it, just by consciously monitoring your mental images and imagining where you want to be.

Combining gratitude for what you already have with present-tense affirmations that allow you to visualize your goal, profoundly improves your results. Focus on these images in the morning when you wake, during the day as many times as you can, and when you lay down to go to sleep at night while it's quiet and you can really concentrate. This will shift the energy you're sending out, and even more significantly, the energy you attract into your life.

You need to know what it is you want and then truly believe you can have it. It's important to set goals and then begin to take action; before you know it, you'll have achieved them. Decide on what you want, then take steps to obtain it with affirmations, imagery and, of course, practical steps. If your goal is to achieve your ideal weight, for example, use your affirmations ("I'm so happy to have reached my ideal weight."), imagine yourself at the weight you're most happy with, and eat well and exercise. Above all, truly believe you can achieve your goal.

Affirmations are so important to this process that I've dedicated Chapter 8 entirely to them.

How Will It Happen?

One of the things that trips people up when they try this visualizing the results they want is obsessing about the "how": How will it happen? What are the specific steps? How long do I wait for proof that it's happening? I say let go of the how. That's the universe's job; that's why you send out the positive vibrations, so the solutions will be attracted to you.

To use the Law of Attraction as effectively as possible to achieve your ideal weight, you can follow these guidelines:

Ask For What You Want.

Imagery is most effective when you're very specific. When it comes to weight, this means imagining what your target weight will look and feel like. This gives you an image of yourself at your ideal weight. One helpful activity is to find old pictures of yourself at your ideal weight and put them someplace where you can see them frequently to solidify this image in your mind. If you don't have any, then look in magazines or catalogs to find pictures that show bodies that look like yours will at your ideal weight, and cut them out. Look at them often. You might even replace the face in the photograph with your picture to help you visualize yourself at your ideal weight. In addition to focusing on this picture, imagine how it will feel, what you will say to yourself and what others might say to you when you're at your ideal weight.

Believe It's Yours.

Believe in yourself in the present tense, not in the future. That is, think of yourself as having already received what it is you want. *Your ideal weight is already yours.* It shouldn't be a hope or a wish, since thinking in the future tense leaves room for doubt. You need to adopt the unshakable knowledge that you've already achieved the goal. You must imagine, pretend, act as if, and make believe that your ideal weight is yours. You must imagine yourself moving through your daily life having achieved your ideal weight. Write out the number you weigh at your ideal weight and place it over the display of your scale, and then don't weigh yourself at all. You may choose to put your scale away, where it can't contradict what you've asked for with your thoughts, words or actions. Rather than focusing on being overweight, change your thoughts to focus on you at your ideal weight and allow yourself to become emotionally involved with them.

Receive With Gratitude.

Living with gratitude is one of the most powerful transformations you can make. It keeps you in a high vibration mode, attracting others, and keeps makes you happier and positive. It's essential to feel as good as possible about yourself while you're going through this process. You can't attract your ideal weight if you constantly find flaws with your body as it is. Emotions are very powerful, and if you hold onto negative feelings about your body, you'll continue to attract more of that emotion and negative thought process. You'll never change your outward appearance if you constantly critique it and find fault with it. In fact, you'll attract more weight. Be grateful and thankful for your body, and focus on all the wonderful and great qualities you possess. As you train your mind to focus on the positive and as you feel better about yourself, you're aligning your mind with the frequency of your ideal weight and attracting it into your life.

Wallace Wattles, the author of *The Science of Getting Rich*, shares something about eating in his book. He recommends that when you eat, you focus completely on the experience. Keep your mind in the present and experience the sensation of eating — chewing, tasting, savoring, and swallowing — and don't allow your mind to drift off to other things. Try this the next time you eat a meal. When you're completely present, you will find that the flavor of the food is incredibly intense and magnificent. When you let your mind drift, the flavor virtually disappears and the body switches to autopilot. If you can eat your food in the present and focus entirely on the pleasurable experience, the food's assimilated into your body perfectly, and your mind is satiated as well as your stomach. This will help you tremendously as you journey toward your ideal weight.

7   *The Power of Positive Thinking*

Meditation is focusing on one thing at a time. Although all the major religions (including Christianity, Judaism, and the Eastern religions) have used some form of meditation for thousands of years, today many people worldwide use meditation outside of any traditional religious or cultural setting for health and wellness purposes. Meditation is an extended and more in-depth form of imagery, and time should be set aside each day to meditate (focus) specifically on your goals.

In meditation, you learn to focus your attention and suspend the stream of distracting thoughts that normally occupy the your mind. This practice results in a state of greater physical relaxation, mental calmness and psychological balance. Whereas the first step to changing negative thoughts or patterns is awareness, the next is practice. You must practice thinking positively, and meditating is a great way to focus your thoughts on positive emotions for an extended period of time. The Complete MindBody FX Lifestyle Program includes a morning and evening meditation practice on CD for you to listen to daily, so you can start and end your day in the right frame of mind. The complete program is available at **www.MindBodyFX.com**.

To get the most benefit from meditation, follow these simple suggestions:

- **Choose a quiet location.** A quiet place with few distractions allows for more focus and less interruption. This can be particularly helpful for beginners. Individuals who've been practicing meditation for a longer period of time sometimes develop the ability to meditate in public places, like waiting rooms or on buses.

- **Assume a comfortable posture.** Meditation can be done while sitting, lying down, standing, walking, or in any other position. Choose what's most comfortable for you and what allows you to focus without physical pain or discomfort, and without going to sleep.

- **Take calming breaths.** Stopping the ever-present train of thought in your mind is much easier said than done. A good way to begin is to take several deep cleansing breaths and think about how your body breathes and notice what it feels like to have air go into your lungs and back out. Relax your muscles from the neck down by consciously thinking about each area and relaxing it. Continue to breathe deeply. This will produce a calm, relaxed state to begin.

- **Allow your mind to fill with positive energy.** Allow thoughts to come and go as you remain positive and relaxed. Consider your life, as it will be when your goals manifest in your body. Imagine even the smallest detail. Release any negative thoughts and practice gratitude for the good that you've experienced so far.

Meditation can be used on its own or in combination with other helpful movement therapies, such as yoga, Tai Chi, and Qigong — a component of traditional Chinese medicine that combines movement, meditation, and controlled breathing. The intent of using these tools together is to improve blood flow and energy flow at the same time.

Practicing meditation has been shown to induce some physical changes in the body, such as modulating its stress response…the "fight or flight" response. The system responsible for this response is the autonomic nervous system, sometimes called the involuntary nervous system. It automatically regulates many organs and muscles, including functions such as heartbeat, sweating, breathing, and digestion. The autonomic nervous system is divided into two major parts:

- The **sympathetic nervous system** helps mobilize the body for action. When you're under stress, it produces the fight-or-flight response; your heart and breathing rates go up, your blood vessels narrow (restricting the flow of blood) and your muscles tighten.

- The **parasympathetic nervous system** regulates what some call the "rest, digest rebuild and regenerate" functions. This system's responses largely complement those of the sympathetic nervous system. For example, it causes your heart and breathing rates to slow down, blood flow to increase to your digestive system, and your body to create new healthy cells.

Meditation works for the physical body by reducing activity in the sympathetic nervous system and increasing activity in the parasympathetic nervous system (decreasing stress and increasing relaxation). This allows your body to respond more fully to the changes you're making in your diet and exercise routine, while also helping you focus your mind on positive thoughts.

Thinking Positive Is A Learned Skill

When I talk about focusing on positive thoughts and energy, I often have people tell me that they're not generally positive people and that it isn't natural for them. I know this comes from their ingrained, subconscious beliefs and habits; although you might think "positive" people are born that way, they aren't. In truth, thinking and being positive are learned skills.

I consider myself for the most part to be a positive person now, but it wasn't always that way. I grew up in a very dysfunctional home, with a teenage single mother. I don't have a single photograph from my childhood where I was smiling. I was so inept at being happy and positive that I had to take workshops to learn those skills. I remember at the age of 30, someone I'd met 10 years earlier told me that it was the first time she ever saw me smile. I spent a lot of time working on myself, to learn to be happy and positive.

You must do things that will encourage you to be more positive and happy; laugh as often as you can; practice gratitude, remind yourself of everything you have to be grateful for; and replace negative thoughts with positive ones.

Improving your self-image, like improving any skill, takes time and practice. Developing good self-esteem involves encouraging a positive attitude toward yourself and the world around you, appreciating your worth while also behaving responsibly toward others. Self-esteem isn't self-absorption; it's self-respect. Thinking positive thoughts about who you are and what you can become is the first step to self-respect. By working from the inside out and focusing on changing your mindset first, you can build your self-esteem; this is what will carry you through to achieving results. The goal of this positive thinking is to give yourself a more positive self-concept, while seeing yourself honestly and accepting yourself, and removing the internal barriers that can keep you from achieving your ideal weight.

I once met with a new client, Mary, who told me a heart-wrenching story. While growing up, she was surrounded by beautiful women: her mother was striking and her sister was your typical prom queen. They were slim, blonde-haired and blue-eyed; even the paperboy would make extra stops at their house to see their beautiful smiles. My client, on the other hand, was brown-haired and chubby as a child. Although they meant her no harm, her family always pointed out the differences between her and the other women of the house. When she and her sister would argue, her sister would call her fat. Her mother was obsessed with Mary's weight and had her on diets starting in second grade.

Not surprisingly, Mary grew up with a very negative self-image and ended up at a staggering 287 pounds. She carried these negative beliefs about herself for 37 years and was still using them as an excuse to remain at her current weight. Her doctor told her she needed to lose weight or diabetes was inevitable, and that her joints were already showing signs of arthritis. Mary finally realized that she needed to let go of these negative beliefs and stop blaming others. It was clear she needed to make a choice to either continue down the road of self-hatred and destruction, or make a conscious effort to forgive herself and her family and start a new way of thinking. It was only herself she'd been hurting all these years.

You'd be hard-pressed to find someone who hasn't suffered some type of trauma in life. Too many of us were raised in alcoholic families; bullied at school; abandoned; or abused emotionally, physically, or sexually. Others have married an abusive spouse or experienced great loss or adversity. Yet at some point, you need to let go of the baggage of the past that's been dragging you down and move forward to a life of hope. You can't change the past, but you can certainly change the future. Wouldn't now be a great time to do that?

I've provided several positive thought strategies to help you overcome negative patterns that have prevented you from achieving your goals in the past. Choose several you feel will help you most and incorporate them into your daily life. Write down these strategies and remind yourself to pause and change your way of thinking each time you find yourself being critical of yourself. As you become more comfortable with each new way of thinking — for example, learning not to apologize or accepting blame for someone else's anger — try adding a new positive thought strategy to your list.

1. **Avoid absolutes and exaggerations.** Correct your internal voice when it exaggerates, especially when it exaggerates the negative: "I always eat too much" or "I'll never lose weight." These are absolutes, meaning they're always 100% true, but there are very few absolutes in life. If you exaggerate or use an absolute, rephrase what you say. For example, "I always eat too much" can be changed to, "In the past, I've often eaten too much. Now, I'm getting better at how much I eat." Then feel good about taking control of your thoughts.

2. **Halt negative thoughts immediately.** Sometimes putting a stop to negative thinking is as easy as that. The next time you start giving yourself an internal critique session, tell yourself to stop it! If you saw a person yelling insults at someone else, you'd

probably tell them to stop, wouldn't you? Why do you accept that behavior from yourself?

3. **Look for the positive.** Did you know that love is a word derived from the Sanskrit word that means looking for the good? Be loving toward yourself (and others), and instead of focusing on what you think your negative qualities are, accentuate your strengths and assets. Maybe you didn't develop enough stamina this month to run a mile, but perhaps your hard work and perseverance led to losing an additional 5 pounds. Maybe you felt nervous and self-conscious when going out to a formal social event, but you received numerous comments from friends that they were happy you joined them and had a good time.

4. **It's okay to blow it.** Maybe you got nervous and embarrassed that you couldn't keep up in fitness class or felt bad that you gave in and ate those potato chips. It's okay. All people have weaknesses, and we all fall off the path at times or don't do things as well as we think we should. Your boss, co-workers, friends, family, mayor, and favorite movie star have all had embarrassing moments and setbacks. Perfection is a high goal; don't start or even end there. Make doing your best your ideal goal. Focus on what you've gained from the process and how you can use it in the future. Avoid focusing on what wasn't done or should have been done differently. Allow yourself to make mistakes and then forgive yourself.

5. **Don't bully yourself!** Don't hold yourself to standards that you wouldn't expect others to meet. It's great to want to do well, but expecting yourself to be better than the best and then punishing yourself when you fail is a vicious cycle. Using expressions like "I should have" is just a way of punishing yourself after the fact. Stop it. Live in the present and move forward. Don't drag the past along for the ride; it gets heavy. Do you remember the children's story of the little train that could? That's how you need to live your life. Keep saying to yourself, "I know I can... I know I can... I can...

I can!" Tell your subconscious you've already done it. Be kind to yourself and remember you can do this!

6. **Encourage yourself.** Instead of focusing on the negative, replace your criticism with encouragement. Give constructive suggestions instead of being critical. ("Maybe if I try to do ____ next time, it would be even better," instead of "I didn't do that right.") Compliment yourself and those around you on what you've achieved. ("Well, we may not have done it all, but we did a pretty great job with what we did.") Giving praise will also encourage others to praise you, and this builds up your confidence to continue on the path.

7. **Lose the guilt.** You're not to blame every time something goes wrong or someone has a problem. Apologizing for things and accepting blame can be a positive quality — if you're in the wrong. You learn and move on. But you shouldn't feel responsible for all problems or assume you're to blame whenever someone's upset. Many of us know people who seem to start almost every sentence with the words, "I'm sorry." I challenge you to remove the word "sorry" completely from your vocabulary. Every time you say, "I'm sorry," you reinforce the idea that you're less than you should be in your subconscious mind. If you're wrong, use the words "I apologize" instead and stop telling yourself and everyone around you that you're sorry.

8. **Only you are responsible for you.** Just as not everything is your fault, not everything is your responsibility, either. You're responsible for you; it's great if you also influence others positively, but you're not responsible for their thoughts, feelings and actions. It's okay to be helpful, but don't feel the need to be all things (and do all things) for all people. This is putting too much of a burden on yourself — and is disrespectful of those around you. Allow others to be responsible for themselves and their actions. You're not responsible for anyone else's happiness. No one can make another person happy; we're all in charge of our

own emotions. Trying to force someone to feel a certain way is just wasted energy on your part.

9. **Be responsible for your feelings.** Just as you can't make other people happy, don't expect others to make you feel happy or good about yourself…and don't blame them if you feel guilty or bad about yourself. You create your own feelings and make your own decisions. People and events may set the stage for your emotions, but they can't dictate them. What others think about you and say to you can only have as much effect as you allow it to have. What's important is what you tell yourself, and how you react to others.

10. **Be kind to yourself.** People often feel perfectly comfortable treating themselves in ways they wouldn't consider treating others. Do you call yourself names like fat, ugly and loser? Would you use those terms to describe a friend? Remind yourself that you deserve to be treated well. Do something nice for yourself sometimes, either in thought (give yourself a compliment) or action (treat yourself to a massage).

11. **Let it go.** You don't need to be all things to all people or please everyone. Give yourself permission to decide you're doing the best you can. Remind yourself when you're doing things well — don't wait to hear it from someone else.

12. **Learn to accept compliments and build your self-esteem, self-image and confidence.** A compliment is a gift to the receiver and a gift to the giver if the receiver really accepts it. The inability to accept compliments is like a plague, helping to create a society of depressed people with poor self-images. Very few people do this it well. Truly taking in a compliment is an opportunity to increase your self-esteem, self-image and confidence. If you don't accept the gift of a compliment, it hurts the giver's feelings and the chance of that person giving you a gift again is decreased.

13. **Let bygones be bygones.** Don't hang on to painful memories and bad feelings, as that's a sure-fire way to encourage negative thoughts and bad moods. Your past can take control of your present

and rob your future if you let it. If you can, forgive past wrongs and move on. This includes forgiving yourself. Forgiveness is done for your peace of mind and your happiness, not for the other person. Forgiving someone doesn't mean you condone their behavior; wrong is wrong. The purpose of forgiveness is to set you free, since holding onto anger is like putting yourself in a jail cell. If you have a hard time forgiving or forgetting, consider talking through your emotions with a good friend or counselor, but try not to dwell on the matter. It's important to work through things, but you can't let the past determine your future.

14. **Focus on what's possible.** Avoid "can't" thinking or other negative language. Don't be afraid to seek help in accomplishing things, but remind yourself that you don't need approval from others to recognize your accomplishments. Focus on what you're able to do. Remind yourself of all your capabilities and positive qualities.

Let go of the past; you must look to the future to change. Stop thinking of old failures. They are the past. This is NOW. Remind yourself that this time you're focusing on the core issues that will ensure your success. ***BELIEVE IT!***

On a separate piece of paper, write down the diet-related events from your past that you feel have been failures. Once you've done that, read it over once out loud. Then, in a symbolic gesture, take that piece of paper and SHRED IT, BURN IT, BURY IT, or FLUSH IT.

It doesn't matter how you choose to dispose of these past failures as long as you do it. You must say good-bye, so long; you're out of my life forever! You choose what you want to say. *In another symbolic gesture, walk to the sink and wash your hands. Now you're FREE to work toward the weight at which you'll feel happy and healthy.*

> *Ultimately, the only power to which man should aspire is that which he exercises over himself.*
>
> **— Elie Wiesel**

8   *Using Affirmations*

To accomplish great things, we must not only act,
but also dream; not only plan, but also believe.

— **Anatole France**

In the world of diet and fitness, positive thoughts are extremely important. Many people have very strong emotions and internal programming that's connected with their physical appearance. Past experiences, either positive or negative, create a stream of dialog that runs through your head constantly. The tone and content of those thoughts are determining factors in reaching your weight and fitness goals. Be aware that it's those past experiences that will cause you to doubt yourself. Release those doubts right now; *The MindBody FX Lifestyle* is different.

You don't lose weight; you release it.

If you've never used affirmations, you might push them aside as something silly. Do you think it's a little self-indulgent to say things like, "I love myself" or "I believe in myself" out loud to no one? You're wrong; it's not self-indulgent at all. In a way, every thought you have and every word you say is an affirmation of some kind. All our self-talk or inner dialog is a constant stream of affirmations. The only reason positive affirmations might seem awkward at first, is that so many of us are so habitually negative in our thoughts and words toward ourselves, it feels strange to say something positive! We're continually affirming subconsciously with our words and thoughts through a flow of affirmations that color our life experience in every moment — making it all the more urgent that the messages be positive.

Your beliefs are learned through patterns you've developed since childhood. Many of these beliefs still work well for you, but others may now be working against you. These dysfunctional beliefs may be sabotaging you from achieving what you want. For example, your parents may have rewarded you with ice cream or some other food-related treat for passing certain milestones when you were young. Though that system of rewards worked and served you in your youth, it set up a habit of food as a reward, which can be detrimental in adulthood.

One way to overcome this embedded behavior is through the use of positive daily affirmations, short positive statements targeted at a specific subconscious set of beliefs, to alter and replace negative beliefs with self-nurturing beliefs. These thoughts and ideas are of your choosing, whereas many of the thoughts and beliefs from childhood were not. It's important that everything you say and think is a positive affirmation. This keeps you focused on your inner goals, and it's a reminder to think consciously about your words and thoughts, and modify them to reflect your positive affirmations.

Almost every self-help program uses affirmations, even if they don't actually call them that. The reason is that they work. The more determined you are to make changes in your life, the better affirmations will work for you. Repeating positive affirmations forces the subconscious into one of two reactions: resistance or acceptance. The bigger the issue you're trying to change in your life, the more likely it is that you'll experience resistance; that is, your own subconscious will "argue" with you when you state your positive affirmations. Conversely, if you experience a sense of joy and well-being as you state your affirmations, your mind is instinctively responding to something it believes to be true. When you feel this emotion, you know your affirmations are working.

Repeating your affirmations with conviction and passion will weaken even the strongest resistance by creating doubt in what was once a strong belief. Doubt weakens the belief, but once the resistance is broken, your subconscious will begin to accept the new, self-nurturing beliefs. The effect can be startling, and things can change very quickly as dysfunctional beliefs are identified and replaced by your own new inner truth.

There are ways to enhance the effectiveness of your affirmations. The more of these you do, as you say your affirmations, the more deeply the message will register in your conscious and subconscious mind.

1. Believe you can achieve them (even if you don't yet know how).

2. Say them out loud.

3. Say them with emotion.

4. Imagine how you will feel and/or look when have successfully achieved them.

It's not a complicated process, nor should it be difficult or seem like work. At first, you may need to put reminders on the bathroom mirror or fridge to focus on what you want for a moment or two each day, but after a short while, it will come naturally and you'll find yourself consistently sending out positive energy — and receiving astounding results from every direction.

If you find yourself experiencing serious resistance or have identified an area of trauma in your life, evidenced by your weight and health, I strongly urge you to seek professional counseling to resolve the underlying issue first. The journey you're undertaking will assist you in letting go of the past, but having proper support around you as you go through the process will make it that much easier.

Because affirmations reprogram your subconscious thought patterns, they affect the way you think and feel about things. As positive thoughts replace negative ones, you'll find that positive change comes easily and naturally. This will be reflected in the results you experience.

As you start out with your personal affirmations, there will be some you love and enjoy saying. These are likely to be very effective for you, and you'll experience changes almost immediately. Others will make you feel uncomfortable, almost as though you're lying to yourself; this indicates resistance, and these areas may take longer to change.

If you find that a specific affirmation makes you uncomfortable, such as, "I'm enjoying life at my ideal weight," when you know you want to release 50 pounds, you can rephrase it, saying, "I'm in the process of achieving my ideal weight." As you get more comfortable, you can switch to the present tense.

How quickly you can resolve a resistant issue depends on the issue, how deeply held the belief is, and how determined you are to bring about change in that area of your life. Your determination to change is perhaps the most important of all. The more determined and prepared you are, the quicker those changes will come for you. Some people make significant changes in their beliefs right away, while others struggle for years. Once you're prepared to embrace and accept a change you believe is right for you, that change will begin to happen.

No matter what aspect of life you want to change, affirmations will make you feel better about yourself and your life. Used correctly, affirmations can change your life, affecting the way you think, reprogramming your mind, and removing the old negative beliefs that have been sabotaging you again and again.

Various studies have demonstrated that nearly 90% of your thoughts are negative. Is it any wonder you find yourself unable to accomplish what you want? Each negative thought or word is a negative affirmation, and these can be even more powerful than positive affirmations, because you often find them easier to accept. You immediately accept the negative as true, whereas you often must be convinced of the positive. These negative thoughts feed and validate your negative internal beliefs. Under this kind of negative bombardment, most people simply don't have the strength to break free of these negative thoughts, becoming hopelessly locked into (usually false) negative beliefs.

Using affirmations is more than just chanting words or phrases. It's an entire process of becoming aware of your negative thoughts and words, and choosing to replace them with positive ones. The more you think of and speak your affirmations, with emotion, the quicker they will work.

Weight and Fitness Affirmations

Since we're focusing on weight and fitness, the affirmations we'll talk about will concern these areas. However, this process will work for any area of your life in which you desire change.

The most powerful time for affirmations is while you're looking in the mirror. Some of the most important messages you've received have come from people who were looking at you while they delivered them. By looking at your face as you state your affirmations, you increase the importance of the message to yourself. You can also see at once any flicker of your own doubt or resistance as you hear the words, see your mouth move, and note your own expression and emotion. This image impresses itself on your mind and makes your words that much more powerful. It also gives you a picture in your mind as you recall these affirmations during the day. You have an image to replay of yourself saying them over and over.

A great way of keeping your affirmations ever-present on your mind is to write them down on note cards or sticky notes and leave them in various locations, such as those I previously mentioned—your bathroom mirror or fridge—as well as your desk or water bottle; you can even record them and put them on your ipod.

To create your own affirmations, begin by taking a piece of paper and making a list of the things that are important to you. Now take a few moments and write out several positive statements for each…in the present tense. They should focus on what you do want, not on what you don't want. For example my affirmations might look like this:

- "I enjoy eating fresh vegetables each and every day."

- "The fresh vegetables I eat every day provide excellent nutrition for my body."

- "By eating fresh vegetables at every meal, I maintain my ideal weight."

Using this exercise allows you to create the affirmations that work for you, not for anyone else. Here are a few examples to give you an idea of how they should look, feel and sound, and start you on the path of creating some that are meaningful to you. Although most of these focus on health, there are also some general life affirmations that are important to include as well.

- "I walk every day, renewing my energy and releasing stress."

- "Walking every day increases my stamina and lowers my blood pressure."

- "Walking every day allows my body to release stored energy, moving me closer to my ideal weight."

- I move beyond limitations and allow myself to embrace change.

- I adapt easily to new routines that enhance my health.

- I nourish my mind, body and soul.

- I choose to allow all my experiences to be joyous and loving.

- I forgive others and myself, release the past, and move forward with love in my heart.

- I love and approve of myself and am at peace with my own emotions.

- I am strong, capable, loving, lovable and perfect, just as I am.

- I am enthusiastic about being active and physically fit.

- My life improves each day and is filled with more energy, vitality, and passion.

- I extend love to people on a daily basis — little by little, task by task, gesture by gesture, smile by smile, and word by word.

- I have wonderful relationships and am happy and at peace.

- I accept compliments from others with grace and gratitude.

- The more grateful I am, the more reasons I find to be grateful.

- I release any fear and know I will succeed.

- I know that I deserve love, and I accept it.

- I'm excited to meet new people every day and embrace my new social life.

- I release any desperation and allow my body to adjust to my ideal weight over time.

- I attract only healthy relationships.

- I'm enjoying being at my ideal weight.

- I choose to make positive healthy choices for myself every day.

- I choose to exercise regularly.

- I believe in myself, and others believe in me, too.

- I express my needs and feelings and reap the rewards.

- I'm my own unique self: special, creative and wonderful.

- I'm at peace.

- I trust in the process of getting what I want.

- I only eat foods that nourish my healthy body.

- I easily achieve the goals I set for myself.

Continued Inspiration

Inspiration is a gift we give ourselves from within that's irresistible and uncontrolled. Unseen creative forces within each of us bring it on. How do we find it? We put ourselves in situations, frames of mind, and the company of others who lend themselves to resounding ideas. **Write a list of people, places, and things that inspire you to reach your ideal weight.** Use these to continually be inspired to stay focused on your goal.

Stay inspired on a daily basis. You may have rolled over in bed, seen a new blanket of snow on the ground or heard the steady pounding of rain on the roof, and had that internal argument of whether or not to exercise that day. Although you have goals in mind, your focus should be on the process. You can't allow your old programming to sneak its way back into your life. You also can't worry about what other people think, or listen to their opinions as to whether you'll be successful or not. Success in achieving your ideal weight isn't a group activity, and it's different for everyone. What works for one person may not for another. Don't worry about the end results, or the how, when, and where you'll achieve them. Don't worry about what others may think. Just stay on course by staying inspired — whether that comes from listening to affirmation CDs, meditating or doing yoga. Discover what inspires you.

Those who understand *The MindBody FX Lifestyle* enjoy directing their subconscious minds to create new and healthy lives. With each new day, they observe the small successes and continue enjoying the process. Before they know it, they're well on their way to achieving their goals. Feed your mind new positive information, and you'll start to enjoy the process as well. As you do this, you create a new habit of thinking; this will be how you create new opportunities in your life that go beyond weight, health and fitness.

Arguments that I often hear when I suggest this new way of positive thinking are reincarnations of the diet excuses. I worked with one client, Anne, who used every excuse in the book, including her baby — who was 14 years old! Many people use the excuse that genetics and circumstances have conspired to stack the odds against them.

Never believe the odds are against you. There will be countless people telling you what you can't do, but why should you rely on their belief systems? How does anybody really know what you can and can't do? They haven't lived your life; they don't know what you may be capable of accomplishing…so how can they set the odds for or against you? They can't. Only you decide what is and isn't possible, and we know that everything's possible. You must believe that. You are capable of achieving anything you truly believe you can, so believe that you can be at your ideal weight, and you will be! As for Anne, once she finally let go of the excuses, she found her ideal weight. Standing tall at 5 feet and 8 inches, she dropped from a size 16 to a stunning size 7.

Calculating the odds makes it seem as though life is a game of chance beyond your control, but it isn't. Odds are irrelevant when it comes to your life and determining what you can or can't do. Think about what you want and focus on the next step without worrying about the end result. Focus on what's going on right now. Enjoy the process.

I know many of you have had setbacks, and I realize things don't always go smoothly. It's very easy to lose faith or confidence in your ability to succeed, but all that's in the past. Begin building your healthy new life by creating a positive belief system, one that will push you to even greater success while you enjoy life every single day. And, there will be plenty of days: healthy living will produce more days to enjoy in the long run by increasing your life expectancy, and even more important, your quality of life.

Anything is possible if you have the right mindset. Once you have that in place, your conscious and subconscious thoughts will create the results you want, day in and day out. Start working with positive affirmations and be inspired, and you'll begin implementing a new mindset that'll allow you to achieve your desired weight — and any other goal you set your mind to.

The good Lord gave you a body that can stand most anything.
It's your mind you have to convince.

— Vincent Lombardi

Creating New Habits

*Great changes may not happen right away,
but with effort even the difficult may become easy.*

— **Bill Blackman**

Achieving your desired weight involves adopting new habits that will help you meet your goal. You often do things repeatedly, trying your best to create a new habit, only to see your efforts fall by the wayside. That's because picking up a new habit takes more than mere repetition. I've provided is a step-by-step list of how to set up a new habit that will endure and serve your quest for your weight and health goals.

Steps To Start a New Habit and Create Lasting Change

If you want to change a habit, and make an everlasting change, the first thing to do is raise your standards. Change the belief and desire you have of yourself in the area you wish to change. Write down all the things you'll no longer accept or tolerate on your journey to your ideal weight, and all the things you want to become and achieve. What do you demand of yourself?

A habit begins with a number of beliefs that together create a strategy. If repeated often enough, the strategy becomes a habit...so how can you change a habit once it's been formed?

It's pointless to raise your standards and not believe you can achieve them; that's called self-sabotage. Once you've raised your standards and decided on the habits you want to change, you must start to modify your limiting beliefs and remove your doubts by following this process:

1. You need to have a firm belief, without any doubt in the achievement and success of your desires. These beliefs need to be like unquestioned commands. They'll shape every thought, feeling and action you'll take. Within the strength of these beliefs lies the "core" to real and ever-lasting change.

2. Your belief needs to be under control. If not, no matter what you decide to change, you'll never have the conviction to achieve your goals or the desire to truly change.

3. Once you have the beliefs that will lead to your success ingrained within you, you then need to have a strategy to achieve the results. I've provided the example result of getting in shape below; follow this strategy to enhance your belief in your goal.

    a. Set your beliefs that you're in great shape and physically fit; you know what you can accomplish (such as running a marathon); and you can see yourself doing this, you can hear the applause (or whatever sound) and you have the feelings. (Don't use the phrase "I want…" as that will result in your goal being pushed further in the future; use "I am…")

    b. Enhance the whole image you've set in your mind.

        i.   Adjust the brightness to bring it to clarity.

        ii. Adjust the color to enhance its brilliance.

        iii. Adjust the size of the picture to make it life-sized.

        iv. If it's a still picture, make it a movie; if it's a movie, make it a still picture. Adjust the speed of the movie until it feels the most realistic.

        v.   If there are sounds, adjust these to make them heard in surround sound.

        vi. Feel the feelings inside you; relishing how good it feels when you can create the body you want.

c. Allow your inner being to do its part in fulfilling your goal – letting change occur. After these changes have taken place and been performed repetitively, a new pattern will develop that will create the habitual change within you.

d. Determine what has to happen for you to know that you've made the desired changes in your life. What would be the final step? Would it be that you can fit in a dress that you purposely bought for a special day? Would it be that people comment on the "new" you? You'll need to write down this final step as your evidence step.

4. Choose several steps you can take each day that will assist you on your journey toward the new you, to make this new pattern ingrained into your subconscious mind and ultimately creating new habits. For the exercise example, your steps might include:

a. Set the alarm clock 45 minutes early.

b. Have workout clothes laid out and the night before, for easy accessibility.

c. Take the dog on your walk; you'll get companionship and the dog will benefit from the exercise, too.

d. Have a healthy lunch prepared the night before.

e. Stock your fridge with healthy snacks you can grab quickly when you're hungry.

f. Plan all your meals in advance.

g. Schedule exercise, meals and other healthy activities into your day planner or PDA.

5. Write down a date when you'll start this new strategy and how often you'll do it. Be very specific. Choose the route you'll take in the neighborhood or which gym you'll visit. State exactly in the present tense what you're doing, as in, "I'm walking three miles today and will do so on Monday, Wednesday, and Friday each week." This is much better than simply saying, "I will exercise each week." Being specific implies a commitment to your goal.

6. Make a commitment to start. Think about what's at stake and focus again on the list you made, thinking about how it'll feel and what benefits you'll receive when you incorporate this strategic change into your life. We've all had the experience of wanting to start an exercise program "next week"; when next week comes and goes, we just put things off, and it never happens. Make the commitment to begin — and follow through.

7. Thank yourself for participating. It's okay to be grateful to yourself; this is a wonderful affirmation. Hearing the words "thank you" relaxes the muscles and deepens the resolve. If someone, anyone, thanks you for something, it naturally makes you feel good. You want to keep doing it to get that praise again, so praise yourself. Soon others will see the positive changes in your life and praise you, too.

8. Notice (without judgment) when you don't follow through. Ask yourself why, but be careful not to beat up yourself over a lapse. Do you need to alter the motivation or the steps to your new strategy? Was there something that created some doubt in your mind? If so, change it back. The results you get are the product of your thinking, so if you continue to be disappointed at what you achieve, you must be willing to ask yourself some hard questions and change your beliefs.

9. Use your affirmations. Often people will take the affirmations they've created and make an audio recording of them that can be played back each morning as they exercise. This is a great way to start the day on a positive and upbeat note while encouraging yourself to commit to your new habit.

10. Journal your progress. This is very important. Journaling is a way to keep track of how far you've come and how much you've accomplished, which can sometimes be difficult for you to remember — a phenomenon we'll discuss in the next section. Journaling can be as simple as a brief paragraph noting what days you performed a certain habit or task and what the outcome was. You can also use a journal to record specifics of your diet and exercise regime as well

as how you're feeling as a whole and any emotional events that are occurring. It's important to do this daily. The more specific you are with your journaling, the better reference tool it will become.

Have a Support System

Most people trying to make changes to their lifestyle or achieve a new goal know that it's helpful for their success to have someone provide support and hold them accountable. Having a "cheerleader" to encourage you is important to your success. If you have a good support system already in place, take advantage of it. You can also find out more information on how to create your own support group in your local community at **www.MindBodyFX.com**.

Can't See Forest For The Trees?

Have you ever made a big change in your life, but soon realized that those around you didn't seem to notice? Let's say you're 20 pounds closer to your ideal weight. You're exercising and getting fit. Do your family and friends (especially your family) start telling you how wonderful it is that you're much slimmer and more energetic? Probably not, because they may be too close to you to see the gradual changes and some may be jealous that you're getting results they're not or disappointed that you're spending some of the time you used to spend with them taking better care of yourself. This can be frustrating, since making major changes to balance your life is more difficult for most people when those changes don't seem to be noticed. It's almost like a void of reinforcement. You expect it to come, but it never does, and this creates stress.

As long as you're seeing the changes, remind yourself that eventually others will see them, too. Right now they may be focusing on other things, like the fact that you're eating healthier and getting up much earlier than you used to. It's also likely that they're busy focusing on their own lives, and haven't even been paying that much attention to every little thing about you. It sounds rather self-serving, but that's really how people function. We like to think we're paying attention to everything, all the time, but it often takes time to notice that something's changed. Often people who haven't seen you for a while will notice first because they haven't been witness to the gradual changes.

How many times have you gone down a clothing size only to have someone ask if you've changed your hairstyle? If you're a parent who "suddenly" noticed that your child is six months old and bigger than a bread box, you understand what this means. You're so close to the situation that you can't see the steady growth; you notice it only in large increments, and even then only occasionally.

If you're going to lead the life you want and be the person you want to be, you must realize that not everyone is watching your progress as closely as you are. You're not always going to find people fawning over you and telling you how much they appreciate your efforts. That kind of reinforcement is up to you. At the same time, sometimes you're too close to see many of your own changes…and you're certainly paying attention!

The solution to this paradox is your journal. As you note the results you see and habits you form in a journal and track your progress, you can quickly see how far you've come. In this way, you can celebrate achieving milestones of health and fitness, even when they happen incrementally. Developing new habits takes concentration and concerted effort, and it can be harder when no one seems to notice or care. This is why it's so important to notice your own progress and congratulate yourself. It may feel good to have someone else remark on your changes, but the best possible situation is when someone else notices something you're already giving yourself credit for.

When you're rewarded for a behavior you'd like to continue, it's referred to as positive reinforcement, something that can work for many behaviors and in many ways. You can give yourself gold stars or write down how great you feel when you create a good health habit; both are forms of positive reinforcement and can assist you in creating the life you desire. When you want to use this technique to strengthen a behavior, it's very important that the positive reinforcement happen immediately, so your mind clearly associates the reward with the desired behavior. If you won a marathon, but didn't receive your medal until weeks later, it wouldn't be nearly as fulfilling.

If there's some behavior you'd like to reinforce in yourself, like exercising three times per week, you can try several methods of positive reinforcement to see what works for you. For example, immediately after returning home from your walk, give yourself praise. Throw your hands up in the air and think, "I did it!" Give yourself a gold star on a chart you see all the time, or give yourself points toward something special — not food, but an activity or other treat. These are very simple, yet effective (and fun!) techniques to keep you on track. The important thing to remember about using positive reinforcement is that it has to be immediate and consistent, and the reward has to be meaningful to work.

Tips For Healthy Living

Here are some tips and suggestions for improving many areas of your life through better health.

- **Eat healthy.** Chapter 11 outlines an eating program that will help you normalize two key areas — digestion and your endocrine system — and help you reach your weight and fitness goals. Eating healthy is such a worn-out and unspecific phrase that for many of us, it's lost its meaning. With all the fad diets that come and go, you may have no idea what healthy is or why certain foods are good for your body and others are downright toxic. To live a healthy lifestyle, you must understand the chemical nature of food and how it works within your body for overall health.

- **Maintain a healthy weight.** Obesity is at an all-time high, and the epidemic is getting worse. Those who are overweight or obese may have an increased risk for diseases and conditions such as diabetes, high blood pressure, heart disease, and stroke. Getting your weight to a manageable level ensures a path to better overall health and energy while adding years to your life.

- **Exercise.** More than 50% of American men and women don't get enough physical activity to provide health benefits; in other words, the most walking they do is between the fridge and the couch. For adults, moderate physical activity for 30 to 60 minutes, five days a week is recommended. It doesn't take a lot of time or money, but it does take commitment to create new beliefs and habits. Start slowly; work up to a satisfactory level and don't overdo it. You can develop one routine, or you can do something different every day. Find fun ways to stay in shape and feel good, such as dancing, gardening, cutting the grass, swimming, walking, playing a sport, or jogging. You'll find some specific recommendations later in this book, such as yoga and weight training, but don't be afraid to vary your routines. Some exercise is always better than none, and once you start moving and experience the increased energy exercise provides, it can be addictive (in a good way).

- **Be smoke-free.** Even though we all know smoking is bad for our health, a large percentage of the population still does it. Health concerns associated with smoking include cancer, lung disease, infertility, and pregnancy and fetal complications. Smoking triples the risk of dying from heart disease among those who are middle-aged. Second-hand smoke — smoke you inhale from others' cigarettes or cigars — also affects your health. If you smoke, quit today! Help-lines, counseling, medication, and other forms of support are available to help you quit, and the health benefits are immediate and substantial.

- **Manage stress.** Perhaps now more than ever, job stress poses a threat to the health of workers and, in turn, to the health of organizations. Balancing obligations can be a challenge, but not taking time for yourself can cause stress overload and burnout. Protect your mental and physical health by engaging in activities that help you manage your stress, such as relaxing, eating healthy, and exercising. Visualization and meditation can also reduce the effects of stress and allow you to react more positively.

- **Know yourself and your risks.** Genetics helps determine some of who you are and what you might be predisposed to in the area of health. Your current habits, work, home environment, and lifestyle also affect your health and your risks. You may be at an increased risk for certain diseases or conditions because of your family history, what you do, where you work or even how you play. Being healthy means doing some homework, knowing yourself, and deciding what's best for you.

- **Treat yourself well.** Good health is not merely the absence of disease; it's a lifestyle. Whether it's getting enough sleep, relaxing after a stressful day, or enjoying a hobby, it's important to take time to be good to yourself. Take steps to balance work, home life and play. Pay attention to your health, and make healthy living a part of your life.

- **Focus on slow and steady progress.** I know you want to reduce weight quickly, but that doesn't necessarily allow you to establish habits that will sustain your new weight over time. When you make overall lifestyle changes, the weight that disappears is much less likely to return. Rapid weight reduction may feel good in the short term, but the results are rarely permanent; that weight usually comes back, and then some. Focus on healthy living and feeling good versus losing weight! **The best way to ensure permanence is not to focus on weight reduction, but rather on a healthy lifestyle.** This will lead you to your ideal weight effectively -- a weight that will be easy for you to maintain. After all, there's no point in losing weight only to gain it back. When your focus is on a healthy lifestyle and not a number on a scale, your desired weight will come!

For a Free Checklist to keep you on track with your goal of achieving your ideal weight go to **www.mindbodyfx.com/checklist**.

Take care of your body. It's the only place you have to live.

— Jim Rohn

10   *Overcoming Emotional Eating*

More die in the United States of too much food than of too little.
— **John Kenneth Galbraith**

Emotional eating occurs when a person consumes large quantities of food, usually high-calorie or junk foods, in response to emotions instead of hunger. Experts estimate that emotional eating causes 75% of overeating.

Many of us learn growing up that food can bring comfort, at least in the short term. As a result, you may often turn to food to heal emotional problems. Eating becomes a habit, preventing you from learning coping skills that can more effectively resolve your emotional distress. Depression, boredom, loneliness, chronic anger, anxiety, frustration, stress, problems in relationships, and poor self-esteem can lead you to overeat...and unwanted weight gain. You refer to what you eat during these times as "comfort" food. Who hasn't sat down to a bowl of ice cream, bag of chips, chunk of chocolate or another comfort food of choice with the goal of feeling better? The problem is, it doesn't make you feel better in the long run, and the results from such comfort food are anything but comfortable...especially when you go to put on your favorite jeans!

Let me tell you about Barbara, who's an expert at losing weight. She should be: she's lost the same 35 pounds over and over again. She's tried all the fad diets, diet pills and diet programs. Barbara's been on the same weight loss/gain rollercoaster for almost 20 years. She diets, meets her goals, and then gains the weight back, each time putting on a little more weight than she lost. At 240 pounds, she fears that she'll soon be over the 250 mark. Ironically, that fear contributes to her eating binges.

Barbara, like many people, is an emotional eater. Food is no longer simply fuel for her body. It has become her drug of choice, her friend, companion, comfort, and distraction from life's unpleasant emotional experiences. At some point, she discovered that eating helps to medicate her pain. That association between eating and easing her emotions is reinforced daily.

There are many different triggers that can send you into a goody binge. For Barbara, loneliness is a common trigger. Having been raised in a family that says, "I love you" with food, she's come to associate eating with love. As a result, when Barbara feels lonely, she feeds her hungry heart. A big meal feels like a letter from home; it's the easiest way to fill her emptiness. Barbara told me that she has to eat bread. It's a must in her life, and something she's not willing to give up. "How else would I feel full?" she asked. The emptiness she feels isn't hunger, but sadness, pain, and frustration; without knowing it, she thinks and feels that bread will fill that void. It's her way of getting the support and the great big, "everything will be okay" hug she craves.

For many people, emotional eating and the resulting weight gain are a symptom of deeper issues. Dealing with any underlying emotions or problems is very important if you want to achieve your ideal weight. As I've already said, weight isn't a function of what you put in your mouth; it's a function of why you eat. It's not until you deal with the subconscious causes and resolve underlying issues that you'll be free to embrace a new and better lifestyle. No matter how much you may rely on denial or escape, the proof of your emotional dysfunction is evident in the extra weight you wrap yourself in like armor.

Take Kara. She eats when she's depressed or bored. Appetite suppressants and antidepressants can mask her problems for a while, but eventually she comes face-to-face with not liking herself and the way she lives her life. Then there's Ron. He has difficulty dealing with his marital problems. Conflict with his wife triggers a fight-or-flight (to food) response.

The situations and emotions that trigger us to eat fall into five broad categories:

- **Social:** eating when around other people. For example, excessive eating can result from being encouraged by others to eat, eating to fit in, arguing with others, feelings of inadequacy around other people, or simply associating certain people with certain foods. Thanksgiving at Grandma's is a good example. How often did Grandma give you a second helping — and because it was so delicious and you felt you had to eat more to make her happy, you ate until you were literally sick? Or maybe your parents made you sit at the table long after everyone was finished because you hadn't eaten all the food on your plate. You were punished for not eating.

- **Emotional:** eating in response to boredom, stress, fatigue, tension, depression, anger, anxiety, or loneliness as a way to "fill the void." Most people have found themselves at a party where they don't know anyone and to keep from running out the door, they make the buffet table their new best friend. The sad part about this is that as you feel worse about yourself and your additional weight, you eat even more. As in the example of Barbara's case, this creates an endless cycle that can kill self-esteem.

- **Situational:** eating because the opportunity is there. For example, at a restaurant, how often do you munch on bread or chips, whether these things really taste good or not? What about that bowl of candy on the receptionist's desk you pass by each day? You might also associate eating with certain activities, such as watching TV, going to the movies or attending sporting events. I often caution people about drinking alcohol, too – not only because it has empty calories, but because drinking is a social activity that inspires many people to habitually munch or graze, not realizing the huge number of additional calories they're consuming. Happy Hour can be devastating to the waistline!

- **Psychological:** eating because of negative self-worth or making excuses for eating. For example, you may eat to scold yourself for those extra pounds or lack of willpower. Have you ever flipped past an exercise show on TV and felt a twinge of guilt…followed by a quick trip to the fridge?

- **Physiological:** eating in response to your body. For example, you might have increased hunger due to skipping meals, or eat to cure a headache or other pain. How often have you gone to get a soda and candy bar when your neck felt stiff or you needed a break from the computer?

Why do you eat in response to emotions? The answer, once again, lies in your mind. You've been taught and conditioned that food's a reward; it fixes problems and heals hurts. Think back to when you were young. Did your parents ever give you ice cream or chocolate to help comfort you when you hurt yourself? Were you ever rewarded with a special dinner at a restaurant when you earned good grades or received a special athletic award? What about high school and college? Did you ever have a junk food marathon as a way to get through the stress of exams? Don't think for a second that this means your weight problem is your parents' or friends' fault. You may be conditioned, but you now make your own choices…so that means you can change.

You eat to reward yourself, celebrate occasions, and entertain others, often allowing food to become the center of social activity. You also eat to calm your nerves and comfort yourself, and you may even use food to numb your heart from emotional pain, hoping it can stifle anger, rejection, or sorrow. This is especially true if you have an unresolved trauma.

Lisa is a great example of this. She lives her life in fear, and it keeps her overweight. As an adolescent, she was raped several times. The trauma of these experiences led her to believe that it isn't safe to appear attractive. By weighing 80 pounds more than her ideal weight, she feels more safe and secure.

She also eludes male attention, which feels threatening to her. Any attempt to reduce her weight is sabotaged by this fear. Any time she gets within 30 pounds of her goal weight, her subconscious triggers her need for protection.

Not all emotional eating has a source this intense, but the results can be the same. If you were raised to think that pretty girls aren't smart, yet knew you were very smart, it could be that you fulfilled that image in your mind and became overweight for fear of not being seen as smart or taken seriously.

Stress also deserves particular attention. More than two-thirds of overweight adults report they eat when they're stressed. When you're stressed out, you may eat extra-large portions or gravitate to junk food, reaching for a bag of potato chips when you otherwise would eat fruit.

Janice is only 10 pounds overweight, but she classifies herself as an emotional eater. Her eating is triggered predominately by stress. As a bill collector who deals with angry people all day, she soothes her frayed nerves at the end of the day with comfort foods. Similarly, Heather often grows angry at her critical, demanding, and unappreciative boss, and she deals with it by walking away — which usually means walking toward the candy machine.

But I'm Hungry!

Emotional eaters will often say they eat because they're hungry and can't seem to control their hunger. Depression, sadness, anger, frustration, and hopelessness are all emotions that can be both cause and effect as the weight creeps on. These feelings are roadblocks to your success. They surface when you see people eating apple pie and ice cream drizzled with caramel sauce, when you stand in line at the grocery store faced with the rows of chocolate bars each seemingly calling out to you, pick me, pick me, or when your family orders a pepperoni pizza smothered with cheese. Oh, the unfairness of it all! How come you can't eat whatever you want? This misery can range from slight to intense, and may require the intervention of a physician or counselor. The feelings can be downright scary, and create a sensation of drowning, or being trapped without a window or door for escape. Begin to manage these feelings by not suppressing them; acknowledge you have them…and begin to understand that emotional eating has nothing to do with being hungry.

There are several differences between emotional hunger and physical hunger, according to the University of Texas Counseling and Mental Health Center:

• Emotional hunger comes on suddenly; physical hunger occurs gradually.

• When you're eating to fill a void that isn't related to an empty stomach, you crave a specific food, such as pizza or ice cream, and only that food will meet your need. When you eat because you're actually hungry, you're open to options.

• Emotional hunger feels like it needs to be satisfied instantly with the food you crave; physical hunger can wait.

• Even when you're full, if you're eating to satisfy an emotional need, you're more likely to keep eating. When you're eating because you're hungry, you're more likely to stop when you're full.

• Emotional eating can leave behind feelings of guilt; eating when you're physically hungry does not.

The particular food you reach for when eating to satisfy an emotion depends on the emotion. According to an article published in the July 2000 American Demographics by Dr. Brian Wansink, director of the Food and Brand Lab at the University of Illinois, "The type of comfort foods a person is drawn toward varies depending on their mood. People in happy moods tended to prefer…foods such as pizza or steak (32%). Sad people reached for ice cream and cookies 39% of the time, and 36% of bored people opened up a bag of potato chips."

I'm sure you'll agree that you probably eat for emotional reasons on occasion. It's when eating becomes the only or main strategy you use to manage emotions that problems occur. Let's face it, if you're feeling a bit depressed, it's unlikely you'll reach for a carrot stick. Since emotional eating has nothing to do with actual hunger, your body probably doesn't need those calories, so they're much more likely to get stored as fat.

It's important to know why you're eating, but it's also necessary to do something about it. Following are a few tips to help you deal with emotional eating:

- Recognize emotional eating and learn what triggers this behavior in you. You can do this by keeping a food journal that helps you keep track of what brings on your craving for certain foods.

- Try taking a walk, calling a friend, playing cards, cleaning your house, playing golf, or doing something active or productive to take your mind off a craving.

- When you do get the urge to eat when you're not hungry, find a comfort food that's healthy instead of junk food, such as a smoothie with fresh vegetables or fruit.

- If you must have some comfort foods, try dividing them into smaller portions. For instance, if you have a large bag of potato chips, divide it into smaller containers or baggies, and the temptation to eat more than one reasonable serving can be avoided.

When it comes to comfort foods that aren't healthy, like fattening desserts, think about this: Your memory of a food peaks after about four bites, so if you only have those four bites, you'll recall it as just as good an experience as if you'd eaten the whole thing. Have a few bites of cheesecake and then call it quits; you'll get all the pleasure with fewer detrimental results.

I'm a Diet Victim!

I can't tell you the number of times I've spoken with someone about a weight reduction and exercise plan, only to hear excuses like these:

"That's great, but it won't work for me, because my husband only wants meat and potatoes for dinner."

"I'm too busy with the kids and my job, and I have no time for exercise."

A diet victim excuse is the line you tell others, and yourself, about why you haven't been successful with your health goals in the past. By and large, this is a conglomeration of misconceptions, assumptions, and denial all rolled up as one. Since I know you've heard or used these excuses at one time or another, let's go over a few just to get them out of the way:

- **"I'm just big boned."** Hmm. Large bones make us tall, not round. The difference in skeletal structure in relation to weight is a function of height. It doesn't account for, nor is it an excuse for, carrying a bunch of extra pounds. You can think of it like a corn dog. If one corn dog is twice as big as the next, does that mean the stick weighs more? Probably not.

- **"My family is big; it must be hereditary."** While certain families do tend to have an easier time putting on the pounds, most often families that are overweight stay that way due to the way they've been raised to think about food, and the way they pass on these perceptions to the succeeding generations. These habits are generally what cause the weight gain, not a specific gene in the family.

- **"My metabolism is slow."** Although a slow metabolism does make it harder to release weight, often your metabolism slows because you've chosen to not live a healthy lifestyle. You might starve yourself all day and then eat a half-pound cheeseburger with fries. This confuses your body tremendously, and it begins holding onto food as fat. If your metabolism is slow, get up and get moving to speed it up. This is one area you have control over, so take responsibility and stop using your metabolism as an excuse.

- **"Healthy food costs too much and tastes bad."** How much do your doctor bills cost? Your blood pressure medication? How expensive will it be to have Type II diabetes due to your weight? Eating well with healthy foods doesn't cost nearly as much as you think it will. Just add up the money you spend on fast food, lattes, and bad habits such as tobacco and alcohol. Learning to eat healthy will actually SAVE you money and increase your life expectancy.

With regard to taste, prepared properly, healthy food can be delicious. Your taste buds have probably never had time to adjust to good, healthy food. Many people who've taken on the challenge of healthy eating and succeeded will tell you that within weeks of eating wholesome healthy food, they couldn't even stand the smell of fried chicken or French fries anymore. The body wants to be healthy and it will actually develop an aversion to fast food if you let it.

- **"I don't have time to cook two meals, one for me and one for my family!"** Of course you don't; no one does…but why would you want to cook healthy meals for yourself, and then continue to feed your family foods that damage their health and establish poor eating patterns they'll follow the rest of their lives? You can choose to give your family the fabulous gift of healthy eating. As I noted earlier, for the first time in history, American children aren't expected to live as long as their parents because of the high rates of obesity and the amount of processed, sugar-laden foods in their diets. Consider that the next time you use this excuse.

- **"I have too much to lose and it will take too long."** This is the perfectionist mindset talking. Who says there's any sort of deadline for you to meet your goal? Eating right and exercising is a lifestyle, not a one-shot marathon! Don't give yourself an artificially imposed deadline that's unrealistic; this will just make you feel worse. Commit to the lifestyle, and the goals will be met along the way.

- **"I'm happy just the way I am."** I've never believed anyone who was overweight who uttered this phrase. Happy people wouldn't treat the only body they have so horribly. I personally am convinced that when people say this, they're really saying they fall into the next excuse category — the worst one of all.

- **"I just can't do it. I've tried and I'm afraid to fail again."** This is the worst excuse people you can use, because it means you've given up. You've convinced yourself that you don't deserve to look or feel any better than you do right now. This mindset keeps more people moving toward a life of obesity and ill health than any other. The only way to ever overcome it is to start the journey toward your ideal weight by focusing on changing your mindset. That's why I'm spending so much time talking about the mental aspect of weight reduction before we ever hint at a food or exercise plan. If you don't have things straight in your mind, no plan will ever work. You must know you're worth it and that you deserve to look and feel as good as you possibly can. Your very life depends on it.

Breaking The Cycle

You have a powerful capacity for healing your body and transforming your mind. To accomplish this, as I've said before, you have to free yourself from the past. When you release old hurts, you grow and learn to recognize happiness, and this helps you stick to your goals and realize your dreams. If the past has been painful, either through diet disappointment or emotional traumas, you must stop reliving it and playing the part of the victim in the story over and over again. Every time you relive a memory, especially a negative one, you keep it alive in your spirit and body. To break the cycle, you have to shed the past story and create the present one. In the new story, you can be determined not just to muddle through, but to thrive.

As you assume responsibility for your actions and become committed to health and fitness, you'll find the solutions. Easier said than done? Well, saying it and thinking it is a good beginning. Every day you have to make a commitment to start with positive thinking. It's neither the win nor the loss that make you triumphant, only the feelings and perception you have regarding yourself. Positive perception and self-affirmation are the first steps to personal empowerment.

There is a Zen story of a great general who was fighting a terrible battle. His troops were outnumbered 10 to 1. The soldiers were frightened, convinced that they would lose because they were physically outnumbered. The general turned to his men and announced that he would flip his magic coin. If it fell on heads, they would fight. If it fell on tails, they would return home. The general tossed the coin in the air and it fell on heads. Believing that destiny was on their side, the soldiers fought valiantly and won.

After the victory, the second in command discussed the event with the general, delighted that fortune smiled on their little army. The general handed him the coin: it was heads on both sides. Because the men believed in their luck, they were victorious...and so it is that we make our own destiny.

In addition to focusing on positive beliefs and eliminating negative self-talk, you need to live in balance. This means eating balanced meals; drinking plenty of water; and avoiding refined sugars, altered fat and processed foods. You need to get eight hours of sleep to reset your biological clock and regenerate cells. You also must do some physical exercise every day to build up strength, stamina and stability. When you exercise, you're an empowered person of substance. You won't feel trapped or paralyzed or allow yourself to be abused, because you've strengthened your bones, muscles, heart, and lungs. A sound mind needs a sound body. By living in balance physically and emotionally, you shed stress. Exercise relieves stress by burning up stress hormones, releasing endorphins, and oxygenating the brain to think more clearly. Exercise also returns you to the present and away from the past...and it's a natural antidepressant and mood elevator.

Living in balance physically, emotionally, and spiritually is the source of energy and joy. Be kind to yourself every day and create personal time and space. If you're too busy, eliminate some of your activities and set realistic priorities. You have compassion for others, even your pets; make sure you also have compassion for yourself.

If you hang your swimsuit on the refrigerator door,
the goodies inside will be easier to ignore.

— The Quote Garden

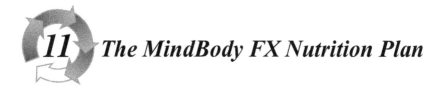

11 The MindBody FX Nutrition Plan

*We can reverse years of damage to our bodies by
deciding to raise our standards for ourselves, then
living differently. Old wounds heal, injuries repair,
and the whole system improves with just a few changes
in what we put into our bodies and how we move them.*

— **Author Unknown**

The key to lifelong health and wellness is finding and correcting imbalances in your mind and body. You create many of your problems through negative thinking, poor decision-making and poor dietary choices. Up until now, you've learned a lot about *your true self* and have been working on resetting your mind to create your ideal weight. Bravo! Now it's time to learn about a healthier way of eating by following The MindBody FX Nutrition Plan.

This is not a diet. Remove the word "diet" from your vocabulary and mind. The MindBody FX Lifestyle has many of the same strategies that you've already used to release excess weight, but it's unique and will mean a new lease on life for you. It's a new way of eating that involves learning more about your body and, ultimately, about what works for YOU and you alone. You'll learn not only the "whats," but the "whens" and "hows" of eating as well. Discovering how particular foods influence your health is powerful information. This plan is distinctive in many ways.

No weighing and measuring foods
No pre-packaged food

No diet shakes or bars
No carb, fat or protein counting
No calorie counting
No constant weigh-ins
No feeling deprived
Tasty and nutritious foods that help you achieve and maintain
your ideal weight

It's time to reset your beliefs around food and your old eating habits and incorporate new healthier ones into your life. Because people naturally want to find anything they've lost, which includes weight, the main focus in this plan is not weight loss…it's to create and maintain a healthy lifestyle. Getting back to a natural state of balance, health, and vitality will help you achieve and maintain your ideal weight permanently.

In previous chapters, you learned how the power of your mind can cause you to become and stay overweight. There are also physiological triggers, such as metabolic imbalances and inappropriate food choices. A metabolic imbalance is a set of symptoms relating to a specific system in the body; these symptoms show that this system is out of balance, so it can't function properly. Metabolic imbalances that contribute to excessive body fat include low thyroid function, poor digestion, low blood sugar, yeast-like fungus, inability to deal with stress, and food allergies and intolerances. Inappropriate food choices vary from person to person, but generally include highly processed foods, trans fats, and refined and artificial sugars.

It's important to realize that we're bio-chemically unique. Just as we have different exterior appearances, we're different inside as well. There's no one else exactly like you, so what works for you may not work for someone else. The ability to assimilate nutrients varies from person to person. People with metabolic imbalances consequently have different needs for certain nutrients and must pay particular attention to food choices or avoid certain foods altogether. However, there are some common threads. We all need some quantities of the same food elements (proteins, fats, minerals, vitamins, water, fiber, etc.). It's important, then, to discover which foods will give you these essential elements, and correct any metabolic imbalances to ensure you're getting the most from these foods.

Given the uniqueness of our bodies, it's no wonder that the "one diet fits all" approach doesn't work. There are many conflicting diets out there: high-protein/low-carbohydrate, low-protein/high-carbohydrate, low-fat, low-calorie and so on. Even among vegetarian diets, there are significant differences: some recommend combining legumes with grains/nuts/seeds at the same meal to consume a complete protein, while others say it isn't necessary. Although every diet has led to a few successes (more often on a short-term basis), there are definitely many more failures. What works for one, doesn't work for all.

The MindBody FX Nutrition Plan is specifically designed to assist in the regulation of your endocrine and digestive systems. Optimizing these two key systems will be instrumental in becoming your best self. Optimizing digestion allows you to better absorb your nutrients. Balancing your endocrine system (the system that controls hormones and emotions) will enhance and regulate metabolic activities, which aid the body in functioning at peak efficiency. The MindBody FX Nutrition Plan also works to safely limit and reduce toxins in the body by eliminating any foods that contain refined and artificial sugars; artificial colorings, flavorings, or preservatives; refined flours or grains; altered fats; and many processed or packaged foods.

The MindBody FX Nutrition Plan uses a customized approach. In The Complete MindBody FX Lifestyle Program, a self-test is included for six of the most common metabolic imbalances that may have prevented you from achieving your ideal weight and feeling great in the past. This is done with a questionnaire that helps uncover imbalances in your system. You then can learn step-by-step solutions that teach you what to eat, when to eat it, and why you're making these healthy choices.

Top Six Metabolic Imbalances

1. **Low Stomach Acid (Poor Digestion).** You require a certain amount of hydrochloric acid in your stomach to be able to break down your foods, particularly proteins. The nutrients from these dismantled foods are absorbed and the waste products eliminated. To reach and stay at your ideal weight, you need to have two to three formed bowel movements a day. If not, the contents of the colon may be held for days, leaving you constipated, overweight, sick and tired. The body cannot absorb the valuable nutrients it needs while accumulating excess waste and toxins.

   Think about that last meal you had. How did your stomach feel afterwards? Did you feel fine, or was there an uncomfortable feeling of fullness, bloating, gas, and perhaps even pain? If so, your system may not be sufficiently processing the food you just ate. There should be none of these symptoms present if you were able to properly digest the meal.

   Poor stomach acid can be due to a number of factors, including high stress, a history of excess dairy and red meat consumption, or age. (Our ability to produce stomach acid at age 40 is half of what it was at age 18.) Your intestinal flora (good bacteria or probiotics) could have been depleted by recent use of antibiotics or by poor food selection, which can also contribute to maldigestion.

2. **Hypothyroidism (Low Thyroid Function).** Undetected low thyroid levels are reaching epidemic proportions. The basic medical thyroid test measures only the amount of thyroid-stimulating hormone being produced by the body. It takes more extensive tests to determine if the hormones are actually reaching and being properly processed by the tissues that need them. The thyroid helps regulate metabolism (the speed at which reactions occur in the body), so if it's not functioning well, every process in the body slows down. Many people with an under-active thyroid also have blood sugar imbalances and digestive challenges. If you've had a hard time releasing weight, are frequently constipated, and wake up tired

in the morning, you should have your thyroid function checked. You can do a quick check at home without a blood test. Take your temperature first thing in the morning, before you get out of bed. If it's lower than 97.8° F (the resting body temperature), you may have an under-active thyroid.

3. **Hypoglycemia (Low Blood Sugar).** Your body requires the concentration of sugar in your bloodstream to be within a specific range at any given time — not too high or too low. If blood sugar drops too low too quickly, you feel a sudden crash. You feel shaky and light-headed, and are often seized with an intense craving for sweets, coffee, or alcohol, all of which bring your blood sugar level up quickly. Responding inappropriately to this craving can put you on the vicious rollercoaster ride of high and low blood sugar. Some sugar is stored in your muscles and liver as backup, but this metabolic imbalance can cause the excess sugar to be converted directly into body fat, creating more fatigue, depression and illness.

    Ideally, when you eat the proper balance of whole foods on a regular basis, your blood sugar remains in its optimal range. When you eat refined carbohydrates (those void of their dietary fiber, like white bread, white flour, white rice, white pasta and white sugar), there's nothing to slow down to surge of glucose into the bloodstream. When your blood sugar gets too high, the hormone insulin is released from the pancreas to remove the excess sugar and take it to your tissue cells. Once in the cells, there are two options: burn the sugar as energy immediately or store the sugar as fat for energy later. Unless you're running a marathon (or have a fast metabolism), your body is going to store these refined sugars as fat.

    Since your body doesn't know how much sugar is still on the way, it sends out excess insulin, which removes too much sugar from the blood and your energy levels crash (hypoglycemia). When your blood sugar level is too low, the adrenal glands release the stress hormone cortisol, triggering the pancreatic hormone glucagon to releases glycogen (stored sugars) from your liver and muscles to normalize it. When this mechanism is employed, your body senses a crisis and thinks it needs to hold on to all fat stores to make it through to its next balanced meal, whenever that may finally be. This up and down of your blood sugar level causes your body to hold on to every stored bit of energy it has available, making obtaining your ideal weight near impossible.

4. **Food Sensitivities (Food Allergies and Intolerances).** In addition to "we are what we think," what we eat and absorb has much bearing on our weight as well. Eating foods that are over-processed, artificially made, too high in bad fats, or void of any nutrition at all will eventually cause your body to break down, leaving you overweight and sick. Take a look in your kitchen cupboard, freezer, and fridge and count the number of boxes, cans, and bags of processed food you stock.

   Food intolerances and allergies can result from the overindulgence in a certain food family. (Too much, even of a good thing, can result in depleted enzymes, decreasing our ability to digest and assimilate a particular food.) Start reading the labels on your packaged and processed foods; notice any similarities? Many packaged foods contain forms of wheat, corn, soy, sugar, salt, and multiple artificial additives and preservatives. When you eat these foods meal after meal, day after day, year after year, your body can become sensitive to them, creating symptoms and intolerances.

   Often a craving or addiction indicates a food allergy or sensitivity. Although people can be born with true food allergies, they can also result from inappropriate food choices — from eating foods that don't assist in having your system function at peak efficiency. One of the many symptoms of food allergies or sensitivities is fluid retention. Discovering and eliminating the food culprits can often result in many pounds of excess water loss alone!

5. **Low Adrenal Function (Inability to Deal with Stress).** Cortisol is a hormone that's released from your adrenal gland whenever you're under stress. This stress can be from life stresses (illness, being late

for an appointment, nervousness about a job interview, screaming kids), environmental (toxins in the air, food or water), or even self-inflicted (starving yourself in an effort to release those unwanted pounds). Low adrenal function is like the shocks in the car that are worn down; when you go over bumps, you really feel it. Like shocks, if the adrenals aren't working optimally, you're more likely to feel and react to those bumps in the road of life.

Cortisol is the red flag that tells your body that you're stressed – under attack or unable to cope in some way. When this hormone is being released in the body, it enters "crisis" mode. During a crisis, do you usually have time to sit down to a well-balanced, whole foods meal? Your body doesn't know when it's going to get its next source of energy, so it will hang on to every last speck of stored fat to get it through this long, stressful period of time. Any time you're stressed, it's not in your body's best interest to burn fat.

How can you tell if your adrenals have been overtaxed? Perhaps you find that something that once caused you little or no anxiety, such as driving, has become a white-knuckle experience. Long-term stress can injure and exhaust your adrenal system. Regulating the adrenal glands, along with eating well and managing stress, can go a long way toward successful weight management.

6. **Candidiasis (*Candida albicans*).** Have you ever wondered why you can't control your cravings? It seems like there's a little voice in your head saying, "Eat the donut! Buy that chocolate bar! Get me some chips! One more cookie!" Actually, it isn't a little voice, but a microscopic fungus known as Candida. It thrives on sugars and starches, so over time your not-so-healthy eating habits have created a nice comfortable place for it to live and thrive in your body. Candidiasis refers to the unnatural overgrowth of this yeast-like fungus, which is normally found in the body in small quantities. The problem occurs when there's a disturbance in your natural flora (intestinal microorganisms) and their environment, so Candida is able to grow out of control, taking over the home of the good

bacteria. If left unchecked, Candida can lead to leaky gut syndrome, an undesirable digestive tract condition that interferes with nutrient absorption and contributes to allergies.

Sugars of all kinds are the natural food for the Candida organism. Since starches have to be broken down into sugars before the body can utilize them, starches also feed Candida. So do alcohol, vinegar, yeasts and fermented foods. Unless your Candida level is brought back to normal, your cravings for these treats will likely continue.

You Are What You Eat

In addition to changing your mindset, there are several good ways to jumpstart healthy eating habits and make you more successful in reaching your overall long-term goal of good health. How would you like to wake up each day feeling better, having more energy and thinking more clearly? Once you rid your body of toxins and excesses, it will naturally start balancing itself, and you'll know this is happening because you *will* feel better, have more energy and think more clearly. With this positive reinforcement, it becomes easy to follow an eating routine to keep your system in proper balance and allow your weight to release easily.

Give your system a chance to help itself. Remove the highly processed foods, refined carbohydrates, altered fats and artificial additives, preservatives, and sweeteners from your diet. Once your body has normalized, you may be able to re-introduce them in small amounts occasionally (e.g., celebrations, when traveling). You may also find that adding a simple-to-make green smoothie once or twice a day will make a significant impact on your health and feeling of well-being.

Elizabeth could not keep her weight down no matter what she tried. She might go down a few pounds here and there, only see them return. She did lose quite a bit of weight when she was much younger, but it all came back. She worked out and was physically active in her daily life; she gardened, parked her car away from the entrance of a store, that sort of thing. She wasn't a couch potato. She didn't even eat potatoes…

yet she struggled with her weight. I coached her using *The MindBody FX Lifestyle* program and nutrition plan, and within two months, she was 13 pounds closer to her long-desired goal. She never felt deprived. By changing her mindset, managing her blood sugar, eating to correct her metabolic imbalances, and choosing to fill her plate with more vegetables, she found the success that had eluded her for years. Her husband and friends noticed and complimented her on the change in her body — and she felt amazing. Today, Elizabeth's at her ideal weight, and plans to stay there.

The MindBody FX Nutrition Plan

This nutrition plan is full of great foods that serve your body well and allow it to reach its highest potential, including your ideal weight. Let's think about what nutrients the body needs to function: carbohydrates, proteins, fats, water, fiber, vitamins, minerals, and all sorts of auxiliary nutrients yet to be discovered or named. All these nutrients have a purpose in the body and they work synergistically: if something is taken on its own, it'll have less benefit than if combined with something else. Consider a whole egg. If you eat just the white on its own, you'll get a certain amount of protein and minerals, but when combined with the egg yolk, you can now assimilate much more protein and minerals by utilizing the fats and vitamins found in the yolk. A whole egg is a complete package.

This brings us to the main principle behind The MindBody FX Nutrition Plan: eat whole foods! Whole foods, like produce grown in the ground or animals raised on a farm, provide all the nutrients we need to survive, and everything we need to be able to use them effectively. Every time a food takes a step away from whole – like in refining, processing, removing this and adding that – nutrients are lost, your ability to use that food optimally is lost, and the food can become a hindrance instead of a healer. If you can't figure out how many steps away from the original state your food is, or how to grow or make it yourself, then it's definitely no longer a whole food.

If a nutrient is found in food, your body will certainly have some purpose for it. Calcium is found in leafy greens, which is great, because you need calcium for bones and structure and to keep your heart beating. Water is found in many fruits and vegetables; that's excellent, as you need water to keep everything flowing throughout your body. Saturated fats – oh wait, do you have a purpose for these? Indeed you do. Saturated fats like those found in animal fats or coconut oil are used to give structure to your cell membranes, and are used to waterproof your cells during times of dehydration. Anything found in the natural food web (that our ancestors have been eating for millennia) can provide nutrients that are required by our body…and the foods that don't are usually poisonous.

It comes down to conscious eating – thinking about each bite that's entering your mouth. Is this a food my body will recognize? Is it benefiting my health and my goals? Does my body have a purpose for it? If you're eating things that your body no longer recognizes as food or doesn't have a purpose for, they become a burden. Energy spent keeping you well and reaching your goals is now being re-allocated to deal with this burden.

Begin to think more about what your great-great grandparents would have eaten, back before processing, refining, packaging, and convenience foods. *The MindBody FX Lifestyle* shows you how to include these more natural, health-inducing foods into your daily regime. By the time you get all these great foods into your day, there will be little room left for the non-foods of your past diet.

Daily Eating Habit Guidelines

We consulted with a leading registered nutritional consulting practitioner to create the ideal way of eating for your MindBody FX Nutrition Plan. Here are the main guidelines to follow and implement into your new lifestyle:

1. **Eat three to six meals and snacks or mini-meals throughout the day.** Keeping your blood sugar regular and within its desired range throughout the day allows for optimal energy, decreases the burden

on your endocrine system, and lets your body know it's receiving a consistent supply of the glucose it needs to survive. If your body receives nutrients on a regular basis, it has no need to store excess fat for times of starvation.

2. **Include breakfast soon after waking.** You've been fasting since last night's dinner, so supply your body with the energy it needs to take on daily tasks without creating stress by running on low blood sugar.

3. **Include a source of carbohydrates, proteins, and fats with each meal or snack.** Each of these macronutrients plays a vital role in your health (carbohydrates for energy, proteins for structure, and fats to protect every cell in your body). Each is digested at a different rate, releasing the energy held within that food into the bloodstream as it's digested. By eating all three macronutrients at each meal, you keep your blood sugar level consistent for an extended period of time, and stay satisfied longer.

4. **Include a vegetable or fruit with each meal.** Produce contains so many health-promoting factors – vitamins, minerals, water, fiber, phytonutrients, and macronutrients – that it's no wonder these foods are considered the best for keeping disease away. They're also generally lower in calories and high in fiber, so you stay fuller, longer for less of your daily caloric allowance. (You don't have to count calories with this plan, but that doesn't mean you want to eat 2,000 calories in a sitting!) Since many guidelines for preventive health include 8-10 servings of vegetables and fruit daily, eating at least one serving every time you eat will get you much closer to your goal by the end of the day. Aim for 1-3 servings of fruit and the remainder in vegetables.

5. **Eat a rainbow.** As much as eating 10 servings of green fruits and vegetables would be good for you, each color group provides a different set of phytonutrients (a plant's defense system) that protects a different part of your body. Eating a rainbow of produce daily will ensure you're receiving full-body protection. Aim to have

a red, orange, yellow/white/light green, dark green, and purple fruit or vegetable daily. You'll be doing great things for your body…and the variety will keep you interested! If this seems a little daunting, aim for 4 or 5 colors daily, and cover all 5 many times throughout the week.

6. **Drink ample water each and every day.** Your body is approximately 70% water. Think of all the ways you lose it – urinating, defecating, sweating, breathing, etc. To make sure you stay 70% water and not 70% mud, drink hydrating beverages like water throughout the day. How much? Take your weight in pounds and divide it by two; that's how many ounces you need in a day. (A 150-pound person would require 75 ounces of hydrating fluids.) Hydrating beverages can also include herbal teas or 100% vegetable or fruit juice (in moderation). Dehydrating beverages (coffee, alcohol, caffeinated teas and hot chocolate) require TWO glasses of water just to make up for the water lost by drinking ONE glass of them.

7. **Eat until you're 80% full.** One of the longest living people, the Okinawans, practice this way of eating. When you eat until you're 80% full, you give your brain time to catch up with all you've put in your stomach. Most time when you eat until you're 100% full, and end up feeling 125% overflowing by the time your brain processes how much you've really taken in. When you're 80% full, it allows your body to be hungry again when it's time to eat in three to four hours.

8. **Live by the 80/20 rule.** Your body is a fascinating organism; it deals with all you throw at it, and yet can still walk down the street. If you focus on eating whole, health-promoting foods in a health-promoting way 80% of the time, then your body can handle the other 20%, when you may choose to indulge in foods that aren't necessarily good for you, but you really enjoy. Again, this is a lifestyle, not a diet, so there's no "falling off." Allow yourself to eat those foods you truly enjoy 20% of the time, without any guilt. (Guilt can create more damage in the body than the food itself!) If you want to fast-

track your way to your optimal weight, 90/10 might be a better rule to follow, but never deprive yourself completely of anything you truly enjoy.

A vital point I want to reiterate is that this is a lifestyle change, not a fad diet or temporary eating plan. This is about balance. The idea is to integrate these changes into your life over time. Many people have trouble changing their beliefs and habits, so to help with this; we've developed a three-phase program: Ideal Beginnings Phase, Ideal Balancing Phase and Ideal Cleansing Phase. We recommend that you make the suggested changes as you assimilate the principles of each phase into your lifestyle.

Creating these healthier habits may take some time, and that's perfectly okay. It's often said that it takes 21 days to create a habit. Keep moving forward and picture yourself at your optimal weight, seeing yourself as you want to look and feel. One idea is to apply a new suggestion from the nutrition plan every day. Once you're comfortable, add another, then another, and before you know it, you'll have successfully created a lifestyle with an eating and exercise regime that's easy to maintain and a natural part of your everyday life.

As stated above, there are three phases of The MindBody FX Nutrition Plan. In this book, we introduce you to the first phase — Ideal Beginnings Phase — to get you used to eating a healthier diet and making incremental changes. Once you're comfortable with this phase of the plan, the detailed version of all three phases can be found in The Complete MindBody FX Lifestyle Program, available at **www. MindBodyFX.com**. In the program, you'll find a complete step-by-step nutrition plan for all three phases to be incorporated into your lifestyle at your own pace. It also includes a grocery shopping guide, daily food and exercise journal, a comprehensive success guide, yoga DVD, morning and evening meditation CD, 7 CD audio program, fitness plans, menu plans, recipes, and more.

Nutritional Plan Guidelines

The following set of food guidelines is for the Ideal Beginnings Phase:

Vegetables

All vegetables are included in this phase, in their whole form and without deep-frying. Keep on skin where possible. Choose lots of variety and colors, and include leafy greens daily. Aim to have at least one serving with each meal.

Fruit

Choose all whole fruit in this phase. Aim for 1-3 servings daily, and include lots of color. Limit 100% fruit juice to one cup daily, and be cautious with dried fruit; it's densely packed with natural sugars and easy to go overboard, so limit yourself to one ¼-cup serving daily.

Whole Grains

All grains, as long as they're in their whole form, can be eaten in this phase. This can mean physically whole (like brown rice or barley), or whole grain flour, pastas, breads, crackers, etc. Sprouted grains are also a great option; the process of sprouting is a form of pre-digestion, so the plant has changed the contents within to a form that's much easier for you to digest and assimilate.

There are more than 500 different varieties of grains in the world, so set your sights higher than just wheat, soy and corn. Amaranth, barley, brown rice, buckwheat, bulgur, kamut, millet, oats, quinoa (pronounced keen-wa), rye and spelt can now be found more readily and can replace your usual wheat products.

To make sure a product contains the whole grain, it's important to read the label. Look for whole grain (including the germ) to know for sure. Whole grain on the front of a box doesn't necessarily mean 100% whole grain; it's important to read the ingredient label to find out for sure. Other names for refined flour include enriched wheat flour, wheat flour, durum semolina (found in pasta) and unbleached flour. Avoid all refined grains that are devoid of their fiber, minerals, and oils; these have become non-foods.

Beans and Legumes

Enjoy navy, kidney, adzuki, soy, black, lima and red beans; lentils; split peas; chick peas; and bean flours regularly. They're a great way to get more vegetarian protein in your diet, plus they're high in fiber. Bean sprouts also excellent – they are much easier to digest than beans themselves and are still nutrient-dense.

Peanuts are legumes, but due to their high propensity toward mold and their extreme ability to absorb pesticides from the soil, the commercially grown variety is not recommended. If choosing peanuts or peanut butter, go for organic to cut down on these factors. Also ensure peanut butter is 100% peanuts; commercial peanut butter can contain a large percentage of added sugars and oils.

A special note on soy: Unfermented soy products, including soybeans, are high in phytic acid, often called an "anti-nutrient" because it removes minerals from the body. Even in Asia, soy is used only as a condiment, not as a primary food source. Processed soy products such as tofu are rich in trypsin inhibitors, which interfere with protein digestion. Research has shown that phytoestrogens (like those found in soy) could be a factor in causing breast cancer, penile birth defects and infantile leukemia. Soy is also one of the most genetically modified crops, and it's goitrogenic, which inhibits iodine from being absorbed by the thyroid gland and can lead to symptoms of under-active thyroid, including weight gain. Fermenting or modern food processing doesn't remove the phytoestrogens found in soy. Fermented soy products like miso, natto, and tempeh, used in small amounts, are healthy options when wanting the benefits of traditional soy.

Meat and Animal Products

There are a wide variety of meat and animal proteins to include in your diet. A good rule of thumb to follow is that if it still resembles how it looked when being removed from the animal, it's the better choice. For instance, a steak is obviously part of a cow, whereas bologna does not resemble any animal part. Choose lean cuts of red meat (preferably pasture raised or organic), free-range poultry, wild game, and wild and freshwater fish and seafood. Eggs should preferably be free range or organic (happy chickens lay happy eggs), and whole; a carton of egg whites is not a whole food.

Avoid those highly processed meat sources: sausages, bacon, hot dogs, corned beef, pastrami, ham, and luncheon meats; all are preserved using nitrates and nitrites – proven carcinogens. Choose wild fish over farmed; there are many concerns with infestations and their impact on wild stock.

Dairy

Dairy used to be a whole food, but now it's pasteurized, homogenized, fat-reduced and fortified, making it a far cry from its original beginnings, and very hard for our body to recognize and utilize properly. A lot of dairy foods are even more processed; how many steps away from whole cow's milk are processed cheese slices? Consider these steps if choosing to include dairy in your diet.

For people who don't have an allergy or intolerance to dairy (though many people do and don't realize it), choose options that are made in a traditional manner, like artisan cheese, whole yogurt, and organic butter. There are beneficial microflora in products like yogurt, kefir, sour cream, and raw milk and cheeses. Read labels carefully; make sure there are no additives, preservatives, artificial colors or sugars added. Specifically in yogurt, look for as few ingredients as possible. Fat-free versions are usually high in artificial sweeteners (toxic to your brain), and removing the fat makes them harder to digest and assimilate. Look for a mid-fat yogurt, sweetened with fruit juice concentrate or other natural sweetener and containing active bacterial culture.

Avoid ice creams, ice desserts, cheese slices and processed cheese, as well as fat free dairy. Some fat is required for the absorption of protein and minerals, so ensure all of it hasn't been removed. Substitute milk with almond, rice, or hemp milk in cereals or smoothies. Avoid relying on soy milk as an alternative.

Nuts and Seeds

Choose a variety of nuts and seeds and their butters to accompany your diet; they're full of healthy fats and protein. Almonds and almond butter, walnuts, sunflower seeds, pumpkin seeds, sesame seeds and tahini, hemp seeds and hemp butter, and flax seeds are just a few of the healthy options available. They're an excellent way of adding protein and fat to salads or snacks. Choose raw nuts and seeds; avoid the salted and roasted versions.

Fats and Oils

Fats are an integral part of your diet; they're required to make hormones and balance moods, for proper brain function, and to make the cell membrane of each of the trillions of cells in your body. Any "diet" that cuts down on healthy natural fats will be followed to the detriment of your health and well-being...and dietary fat does not equate to adipose (stored) fat. Eating healthy fats doesn't make you fat. Again, if a fat comes from a natural food, your body knows what to do with it and has a purpose for it. Your body even requires saturated fats; they add great stability to cell membranes and work as waterproofing when you're dehydrated.

Recommendations for fat and oil use:

- For high heat/stir fry: coconut oil, animal fats, and ghee (clarified butter)

- For medium heat: butter, sesame oil, and grape seed oil, in addition to those above

- For low heat: extra virgin olive oil, in addition to those above

- For salads (no heat): avocado oil, almond oil, pumpkin seed oil, walnut oil, unrefined flaxseed oil, hemp seed oil and hazelnut oil, in addition to those above

Additional great fat sources include avocadoes, olives, coconut milk, nuts or seeds and their butters, and fish.

Cut out all hydrogenated, partially hydrogenated and trans fats, and any industrially processed oils such as soy, safflower, cottonseed and canola oils. This also includes margarine and vegetable shortening. Read your vegetable oil label; does it say what vegetables are used? Avoid all fried foods.

Beverages

Water is always the beverage of choice, preferably filtered in some manner. Add lemon and sea salt to increase pH and make it more palatable if necessary. Choose other hydrating beverages like herbal or decaffeinated teas, unpasteurized or freshly juiced vegetable and fruit juices, and green or white teas (which contain some caffeine, but have great health benefits).

Reduce caffeinated, alcoholic and carbonated beverages. Beverages to avoid completely include soft drinks, diet soft drinks, sport drinks, fruit punch, ground commercial coffee, and sugar-laden or sugar-free lattés and other café drinks. When wanting to release weight, remember not to drink your calories! Unless you're having a smoothie as a meal or snack, there's no real need to include extra calories from drinks.

Sweeteners

Again, think of steps away from whole. Natural sweeteners like unpasteurized honey, maple syrup, agave nectar, molasses, sucanat, brown rice syrup and fruit concentrates can all be used in moderation. Stevia is a plant that tastes 300 times sweeter than sugar, and makes a good substitute without adding any calories. A great tip is to substitute half the required sugar for something like honey or maple syrup, and the other half with the equivalent amount of this herb (remembering that one cup of sugar equals one teaspoon of stevia), as on its own it can be slightly bitter.

Avoid completely all artificial sweeteners and reduce greatly your refined sugars, including brown sugar, cane sugar, corn syrup, fructose, fructose-glucose, high-fructose corn syrup, sucrose, maltose, maltodextrin, dextrose, and corn sugar. Some of these sugars are fine when they're found naturally in a food (like fructose in fruits), but when removed and refined they cause major imbalances in your body.

All artificial sweeteners are detrimental to your health for many reasons. Many are neurotoxins (poisonous to the brain) or are highly toxic to other systems in your body. They're used to reduce calories by replacing fat (therefore not contributing to your good brain and emotional health) or natural sugars (which you use as fuel). When your body tastes the sweetness of an artificial sweetener, it's expecting glucose and prepares for it. A release of insulin removes the glucose from your bloodstream in anticipation. When it doesn't arrive, low blood sugar can result. As well, your body thought it was getting sugar and didn't, so it craves more and more food until it's satisfied, causing an increase in appetite and eating. Think about it; if artificial sweeteners did what they claimed to do, would we be facing our current obesity epidemic?

Non-Foods

A few other foods are so far removed from a whole food (or were produced in a lab) that they can't even be included in the above categories; they are non-foods and therefore have no role in your body...and no role means a big burden on your system. Avoid all highly processed, packaged, refined food containing additives, preservatives, artificial colors, sweeteners, flavors, and any other type of enhancer. Anything claiming to be low fat or low calorie (unless it's broccoli) has had something removed and more than likely something added back in. If when reading your ingredient label a) you get bored because the list is too long, b) you cannot pronounce an ingredient, or c) think you're reading the inventory for a chemistry lab, then put that non-food anywhere but your mouth. An even better idea is to eat foods that don't require a label – they are what they are.

Phase 1 – Ideal Beginning Phase

Day 1

BREAKFAST

Very Berry Smoothie (see recipe)

SNACK

Rye crackers with almond butter, peach

LUNCH

Chicken and avocado in a sprouted grain wrap, homemade vegetable soup

SNACK

Cut-up vegetables of your choice (radish, bell pepper, snow peas, carrots, tomatoes, etc.) with hummus or pumpkin seeds

DINNER

Wild prawns, brown rice, steamed broccoli and cauliflower, and green beans sautéed in butter and garlic

Note: The MindBody FX Nutrition Program can easily be adapted for vegetarians or vegans.

VERY BERRY SMOOTHIE

Approximately 1 cup of fruit – various berries or whole fruit; whatever is in season

¼ to ½ cup (or more) filtered water

2 scoops protein powder (flavor of your choice)

1 tsp – 1 tbsp unrefined flaxseed oil

Ice cubes

Place fruit in blender. Add filtered water and ice cubes. Blend until smooth. (Add more or less water for desired consistency.)

Add protein powder and flax oil at the very end, and mix for no more than a few seconds to avoid overheating the amino acid profile of the protein and degrading the oil. Pour contents into a glass and enjoy!

For variation and extra functional nutrition, try adding any of the following ingredients:

*Ground flaxseeds, 1 tbsp. *Flaxseed oil, 1 or 2 tsp. *Cinnamon, to taste *Nuts and seeds (raw or in a nut/seed butter form) *Wheat or oat germ, 1 tbsp. *Green foods powder, 1 or 2 scoops *A squeeze of lemon or lime juice *Handful of dark leafy greens (spinach, Swiss chard, collards or kale for added nutritional value)

Getting Started

To help you get started, here's a list of healthy living tips to keep you on track in The MindBody FX Nutrition Plan. Start with the Daily Eating Habit Guidelines from earlier in this chapter and add these 10 tips to ensure they become habits for life-long wellness.

1. Avoid the refined whites: white sugar, white flour, white rice, white pasta and white bread. These are the foods that spike your blood sugar and cause insulin to store the excess as fat. They're also responsible for mood swings, headaches and shakiness. There are whole food options for all of these; read all labels and always make conscious whole foods decisions.

2. Eliminate fried food or foods cooked in heated oils from your diet (besides the healthy fats and their temperature ranges listed above). It's amazing how often we choose fried food, even when there are healthier choices, e.g. it's just as easy to steam veggies or stir-fry them with coconut oil rather than frying them in harmful oils. In a short period of time, you'll actually develop an aversion to even the smell of fried food and your stomach won't let you eat much of it, either; it can make you feel ill.

3. Think about the origin of your food. Is it coming from a farm down the road or from a factory on the other side of the world? Fresh food

loses its nutrient content as it travels to your table; has it been picked yesterday or three weeks ago? This also makes us think seasonal; when is that food actually supposed to be available in your climate? We all know that a peach in January just doesn't taste the same as one straight off the tree in the summer. Shop at farmers markets and stands, use fresh food delivery services, and source out foods that are grown in your geographical area when the season allows.

4. To ensure a rainbow in your diet, ensure a rainbow in your shopping cart. If a rainbow of produce is in the fridge or on the counter, you're obviously much more likely to eat it than if it wasn't there at all! Find ways to add a variety of color to your plate by eating rainbow stir-fries, chili, soups or smoothies.

5. Choose organic when possible. These are foods that haven't been contaminated with chemicals like pesticides, drugs, or added hormones; are grown under fair labor and good farming practices; and cannot be genetically modified. Organic foods have to be strong to defend themselves from pests naturally – these "superpowers" (and a higher level of nutrients) are passed along to help build your own defense system.

    It's great to know all these benefits, but it's sometimes hard to put into practice. Spend your time and produce dollars on organic versions of the "dirty dozen": peaches, apples, bell peppers, celery, nectarines, strawberries, cherries, kale, lettuce, imported grapes, carrots, and pears. These are the most contaminated produce on the market, so switching to organic is the best bet for your buck...and health. Also choose organic meat, dairy, eggs, and butter, as toxins are stored in the fat cells of animal foods.

6. Read the ingredient label of every food before you buy. The marketing label entices you and the nutrition facts give some numeric values, but the real dirt is in the ingredient label. Items are listed by proportion in the product. Again, read the list; can you recognize each ingredient? Do you know how these ingredients were made? Can you pronounce each name? Is the list so long that you're

bored by the end? Is this something you want to put in your body? These are all questions to ask before a food ever goes into your cart. Compare your options and make the best choices available to you.

7. Eliminate processed foods from your diet. This includes processed dinners, pizzas, junk foods and fast food (burgers, fries, cakes, pastries, candy, chocolate, donuts, etc.). This is one of the hardest things to do for most people, not because we aren't aware that these foods are less than great on the nutritional scale, but because snacking on junk foods may be deeply ingrained in our daily habits. It's also ever-present in our awareness, thanks to the marketing efforts of large companies. We're surrounded by businesses offering cheap and convenient junk food, and bombarded by advertising enticing us to nibble constantly. Cheap and convenient does not equate to health promoting.

8. Use a plate or bowl to visually see your portions. Eating directly out of the box or package can easily lead to overeating. When you don't set aside a portion, that small handful of pretzels quickly becomes two, then three, and so on. Take time to put a serving of food on a plate or in a bowl. Eat that portion and only that portion. Many people find it very useful to use a small plate when they eat meals; a small plate covered with healthy dinner selections seems like a lot of food, but a large one covered containing the same amount of food seems like an appetizer. When your brain sees that the small plate is full, it will be completely satisfied.

9. Don't feel you have to clean your plate when you eat out. Many restaurant meals are extremely super-sized, but so nicely presented that it's hard to notice just how much extra food is on your plate. As much as it may be ingrained, never feel like you have to finish everything. Stop when you're 80% full, even if there's enough left to take home for tomorrow's lunch or only two bites. This food does more than just going into the garbage if you eat it instead; it either goes to waste or to your waist! Don't use your body as a garbage disposal.

10. Chew your food well, eat slowly, and pay attention to it. Chewing is the first stage of digestion (and there are no teeth in your stomach!) and also allows the body time to recognize when it's satisfied. If you eat very quickly and barely chew, your body doesn't have as much time to send the signals to your brain telling it you're full, and it becomes very easy to overeat. Eat your food with your eyes and nose as well as your mouth; enjoy your food with all your senses to get the most out of it, a habit the French have mastered well.

With this plan, you have the keys to a lifetime of healthy eating. I haven't asked you to cut anything completely out of your diet. I may strongly recommend you avoid certain foods, especially if you want to release weight or if you have a metabolic imbalance to correct. But even within these recommendations, I try to suggest alternatives. Although I want you to be successful in achieving your ideal weight, I also want to teach you to make the best choices for the foods you'll eat. Switching from white rice to brown, white breads to sprouted-grain breads, eggs and bacon to eggs and veggies, refined sugars to maple syrup and fruit...all these should be a goal with this plan. Remember that your subconscious will seek out what it thinks you've lost, so if this plan simply prohibited sugars, it wouldn't be long before your body would crave it in any and every form, good or bad. I'd rather give you healthy alternatives with no deprivation.

If adopting a new habit each day from The MindBody FX Nutrition Plan was all you had to do to overcome your ideal weight obstacles, wouldn't you do it? You'd think twice when faced with the choice between a salad topped with nuts and a fat-filled, sodium-laden "mystery meat" sandwich. In the cafeteria line, you'd make sure to include a good serving of green vegetables or salad along with that meatloaf surprise. You might find it easier to pour yourself a cup of herbal tea instead of that second cup of coffee, or keep a water bottle with a squeeze of lemon in it on your desk. Fortunately for you, it's that simple! Remember to take these kinds of small steps, and know that achieving and maintaining your ideal weight is a lifelong process that involves creating a healthy lifestyle to manage it. Your goal in following The MindBody FX Nutrition Plan will be to create these healthier habits so they last a lifetime…and never end up in an excess weight situation again. What you put into your mouth and how you treat your body, in combination with your mindset, are the keys that will unlock the door to your success in reaching your ideal weight.

For a Free Special Report on Toxins and Excess Weight and how you can reduce the amount of toxins in your body to shed weight faster and easier go to **www.mindbodyfx.com/specialreport2**.

My advice is to go into something and
stay with it until you like it.

— Milton Garland

The Importance of Water

Your body is the baggage you must carry through life.
The more excess the baggage, the shorter the trip.

— Arnold H. Glasgow

Your body is mainly made up of water – around 70% give or take, depending on your age, gender and health. Water makes up most of the fluids in your body: blood, lymph, digestive juices, urine, tears and sweat. It's involved with almost every bodily function: circulation, energy production, digestion, absorption, and elimination, and carries the electrical current that allows your heart to beat, your muscles to contract and your brain to think. Are you paying attention to your level of hydration?

You lose water daily through urine, feces, sweat, breathing and your skin. You get water daily through beverages, food and metabolism. The loss and gain of water in your body needs to remain equal to prevent dehydration. As your body becomes dehydrated, systems start to shut down and revert to back-up modes of function. At a 2% reduction of body weight in fluids, you'll be thirsty. At 4%, your muscles will have a significant drop in strength and endurance. At 10-12%, heat tolerance is decreased and you'll feel very weak. If your body gets to a 20% reduction of body weight in fluids, you may lapse into a coma and die.

Blood circulates and deposits water in the sweat glands, kidneys and lungs. Blood collects new water supplies from the bowel if it doesn't have enough to flow properly, taking away from the water required for proper bowel movements; this is a major cause of constipation. If there's still not enough available, the water volume of the blood drops, making the blood thicker and impeding circulation. When your circulation slows, your brain doesn't get all the nutrients or oxygen it requires as quickly as it should, which can result in the following reactions:

- You may reflexively yawn in an attempt to get more oxygen.

- You may crave sweet foods, which is your body's attempt to increase blood sugar and therefore energy.

- You may feel drowsy, since during sleep less oxygen is required for the brain.

There are numerous smaller health complaints that you may experience that can be eliminated or reduced simply by drinking water. Below are just a few of the specific roles of water:

- Water is essential for the body to sweat and therefore release toxins. Sweat helps to cool the body during exercise or hot weather. You may lose up to 32 ounces (1 liter) of water during exercise, so it's very important to stay well hydrated while working out.

- Water allows for more efficient cellular repair. As cells are routinely damaged, water may assist with swift healing, plumping and repair.

- Water is required as part of your stool to allow it to flow out of your body. When dehydrated, there's insufficient water to remove waste and toxins two to three times daily via stool.

- Water lubricates the joints and lessens discomfort from arthritis or back pain. It also decreases the likelihood of having arthritis.

- Water allows red blood cells to carry oxygen more efficiently, resulting in better muscular function and increased mental acuity.

- Water helps the blood cleanse toxic waste from various parts of the body and carries it to the liver and kidneys for removal.

- Water decreases stress, anxiety and depression, and allows the brain to function normally.

- Water restores normal sleep patterns and helps decrease the incidence of insomnia. (Initially, you may find your sleep interrupted with regular nocturnal trips to the bathroom, but that will pass...no pun intended.)

- Water prevents fatigue and drowsiness.

- Water slows down the aging process and makes the skin smooth.

- Water decreases premenstrual pains and hot flashes.

- Drinking water allows you to distinguish between the sensations of thirst and hunger, so you only eat when you're actually hungry, which aids in weight reduction.

- Water diminishes morning sickness during pregnancy or nausea in general.

- Water prevents the loss of memory as you age.

- Water lessens addictive urges, including those for caffeine, alcohol and some drugs.

Here are some other important and interesting facts about water:

- 75% of Americans are chronically dehydrated.

- A weak thirst mechanism is mistaken for hunger by 37% of the population.

- Mild dehydration slows metabolism.

- A University of Washington study discovered that one glass of water stopped hunger pangs for almost 100% of the dieters it studied.

- Wanting an afternoon nap is likely triggered by lack of water.

- Research shows that 8 to 10 glasses of water per day will significantly reduce back and joint pain.

- Feeling a bit fuzzy headed? Reach for water. A slight drop in dehydration can trigger mental fogginess.

- Research shows that five glasses of water a day have a positive effect on slashing cancer rates.

- Water is the best way to combat water retention. Too little water and your body thinks it's in a drought situation and reserves as much as it can.

- Water helps burn fat more efficiently. If the kidneys aren't working well, the liver must help them, which takes it away from one of its many other functions: burning fat.

- Dehydration taxes the heart by causing it to pump faster to get sufficient oxygen to your muscles.

Not only is it important to drink enough water, it's also crucial to drink the right kind of water. You hear on the news almost on a daily basis about the impurities dissolved in tap water. There's been much discussion over the past few years about water quality, and the effect that it may have on health. Many health experts believe that low quality tap water can pose health concerns, particularly if it's relied on as your main source of water.

These health concerns have made millions turn to bottled water, with the assumption that it's of better quality. Unfortunately, some bottled water is often just tap water in a pretty container.

To get the most benefit from the water you drink, it's important to understand that most water is slightly acidic. Pure distilled water has a neutral pH of 7.0, and most other water falls slightly below that number. Alkaline water is especially good for your body. As the majority of the foods you eat create acid wastes in your system, it's healthy to drink alkaline water (with a pH higher than neutral) to counterbalance this process. Slightly alkaline water helps to neutralize acids and remove toxins from the body. To increase the alkalinity of your water, add a slice of lemon or fresh lemon juice and a pinch of sea salt to each glass. Tasty and healthy!

When you think about increasing the quality of your drinking water, you naturally think of water filters that are readily available at your local discount store. Make no mistake; these handy and affordable filters go a long way toward making your drinking water more beneficial and healthful. However, if you're looking for life-giving, energy-boosting nourishment from your drinking water, they only really scratch the surface.

Transforming your water from something that simply quenches your thirst to something that you crave due to the energy and vitality it gives you isn't a complex or difficult process. You can greatly increase the quality of your drinking water using one of the following:

Home Water Distillers. Water distillers heat tap water electrically to the boiling point. The purified condensation then drains into a clean container, leaving all the impurities behind in the boiling chamber. Distillation kills and removes bacteria, viruses, cysts, and heavy metals. Although there's debate about whether distilled water removes beneficial minerals along with disease-forming metals and microorganisms, it's useful to note that the mineral content in water is so minute that you'd have to drink approximately 600 eight-ounce glasses to attain the RDA of calcium and 1,800+ glasses to fulfill your daily requirement of magnesium. Distilled water also has more oxygen ions and fewer hydrogen ions, making it far less acidic and more alkaline than some other types of water.

Osmosis Water Filters. Reverse osmosis utilizes a fine, semi-permeable membrane to filter water, a process known as hyper-filtration, which removes bacteria, salts, sugars, proteins, particles, dyes, and other damaging elements. This allows the water to pass through, while the contaminants are removed and held in the membrane. In the majority of reverse osmosis filters, this membrane is self-cleaning, allowing for the purest water to be provided. Reverse osmosis units can use as little as two or as many as 10 gallons of water to make one gallon of pure water. As with distilled water, reverse osmosis water is far more alkaline than tap or bottled water.

Water Ionizers. Water ionizers electrically enhance water by running it across positive and negative electrodes to ionize it, separating it into alkaline (70%) and acidic (30%). This is exceptionally beneficial, as the alkaline water is used for drinking, while the acidic water can be used on the outside of the body, as it's proven to kill many types of bacteria. The quality of ionized water is reputed to surpass water from any other source. For instance, ionized water is the only type of water that has a low surface tension, which allows for greater absorption of water and nutrients into your body. Some water ionizers also come with an alkalinity adjustment setting that allows you to set your preferred level of alkalinity. This is an incredibly useful benefit, one I recommend you get if you decide to purchase a water ionizer, to obtain the highest quality of alkaline water.

Hydrate...or Suffer the Consequences

Most North Americans don't drink nearly enough water. Not only that, they often drink beverages that actually dehydrate the body, such as coffee and alcohol. Water hydrates the body and helps all your bodily functions perform better. When you're dehydrated, you can experience headaches, irritation and difficulty concentrating. Dehydration has also been shown to slow metabolism and make you retain the little water you're taking in. In other words, not drinking enough water makes it much more difficult to achieve your ideal weight.

By the time you experience thirst, your body is already very dehydrated. Know what your body requires and sip water regularly throughout the day. A good practice is to keep a large stainless steel water bottle with you during the day in your car, on your desk or on your kitchen counter. Make it a goal to drink at least two to three full bottles before you get to your evening meal. This will ensure minimum daily hydration.

As you hydrate your body properly, you'll develop more of a thirst for water. We often misinterpret thirst for food cravings, so you might already have more of a thirst than you realize. Drinking water should be one of the first things you do in your quest for good health. Since it improves the function of your body as a whole and increases your metabolism, it actually helps you reduce unwanted pounds.

It's ideal to take in a good portion of your daily water requirement as soon as you get up in the morning. This flushes the metabolic wastes created as the body worked in your sleep, and provides your body and mind with the best start possible for the day.

If you're someone who doesn't drink much water, you might start by adding a glass in the morning and one between each meal. Eventually, you'll be able to progressively increase your water consumption to 8-10 glasses per day. This will allow your body time to become accustomed to the elevated water intake. Often during these first few weeks, you may be tempted to stop drinking because you feel like the water is running through your system within minutes. It's important to be consistent and stick to your plan. Your body needs time to balance out the new intake level and get used to being able to function with enough water when it had to hoard it in the past. Adding a pinch of sea salt to your glass will also normalize the bathroom trips by allowing the water to enter your cells and not just your bloodstream. People who dramatically increase their water intake will often reduce five to seven pounds in the first week. They feel better and more energetic, experience a reduction in appetite and have noticeably clearer skin. Yes, skin eruptions can be a sign that you're a toxic waste dump inside!

Dehydration is one of the biggest reasons you experience cravings for junk foods, or foods loaded with sugar and/or salt. Being well hydrated lessens those cravings. If you don't like drinking just plain water, add some fresh lemon juice or a slice of lemon to it.

Here are a few more ways to drink more water and stay hydrated:

- Make water your top beverage choice.
- Start your day off with a glass of water before breakfast.
- Have a glass of water between each meal and snack.

- Take water with you when you go shopping, to sports events or to exercise.

- Choose water over other beverages in social situations.

- Make a conscious decision not to drink your calories.

- Switch coffee to Swiss-water decaf, black tea to rooibos tea, and colas to juice or water…to decrease the amount of water you're losing.

It's important to develop a plan on how to add more water to your daily regime. Water is so very important to your health and well-being that you must focus each day on drinking the required amount. It's so important that without it you would die. The same can't be said of French fries, ice cream or chocolate.

Clogged with yesterday's excess,
the body drags the mind down with it.

—Horace

13 *The Value of Supplements*

The time for action is now. It's never too late to do something.
— **Carl Sandburg**

Consider for a moment all the beating and abuse your body has taken over the years. Scary, isn't it? The first huge step to correcting this is to adopt The MindBody FX Nutrition Plan, providing your body what it needs and eliminating what it doesn't. This is great for not doing any additional damage, but what can you do to reverse some of the previous damage and get rid of the previous garbage that's being stored in your body from when you weren't so aware of what you were doing? Supplements are an excellent tool to help you regain full balance in your body. They can provide nutrients you're lacking, pull toxins out of your body, and allow you to digest properly to attain the most benefit from your food.

You can't live off supplements alone; they're meant to "supplement" a whole foods diet. Think of them more as an insurance policy for your body. They won't protect you if you eat junk food all the time, but they're a bit of coverage for those days when you consciously choose to eat non-foods. Just as you have insurance for your car, house or yourself, consider taking out a policy for your body and health with the appropriate supplements.

You'll find many, many supplements exist when you start investigating them. The ones I mention in this book are those I find most beneficial for weight release and correcting metabolic imbalances. If you're taking medications, or you have a history of intolerance to supplements, it's probably a good idea to check with your physician before embarking on a supplement program.

Digestive Aids

You can't be truly healthy without adequate digestion, assimilation and elimination. Nutritional researchers have now shown that the underlying cause of many health symptoms is autointoxication, which occurs when certain toxins are re-circulated back into your bloodstream, slowly poisoning your body, due to poor elimination. This explains why it's essential to your health to have two to three bowel movements per day rather than have waste staying for days in your digestive tract.

Nutrients aren't being properly absorbed from foods or supplements if you're experiencing poor digestion. Your body needs to produce enough hydrochloric acid and other enzymes to properly break down proteins, fats, and carbohydrates. Low hydrochloric acid levels and enzyme deficiencies may also impair your immune function, resulting in illness.

As noted earlier, you have half the ability to produce hydrochloric acid at age 40 as you did at age 18, which suggests that as you age, you're more likely to require some type of digestive support. Look for a digestive aid supplement that contains hydrochloric acid (to begin the breakdown of proteins) and bile (to begin the breakdown of fats) as well as a full spectrum of enzymes. Hydrochloric acid and bile also destroy gastrointestinal parasites. Taking digestive enzymes won't suppress your own ability to produce enzymes; after eating a meal, wait a few minutes and then take your supplemental enzymes to give your body's natural enzymes a head start and allow the supplement to work above and beyond what your own body can handle.

Probiotics (Good Bacteria)

Healthy bacteria are natural microorganisms that assist in keeping your immunity strong and improve digestion by stimulating peristalsis.

Friendly bacteria help produce good lactic acid to help maintain the integrity of the large intestine. They also produce some B vitamins and vitamin K, and are involved in the breakdown of the remaining proteins and fatty acids to their smaller components.

Unhealthy bacteria do the opposite—they weaken your immunity and hinder digestion—which helps promote disease. Non-foods such as processed foods, hydrogenated fats, and refined sugars contribute to the imbalance, as they feed these unhealthy bacteria. The typical North American diet today consists largely of these non-foods.

Having well-functioning digestive flora is important to continued good health. It all starts with the colostrum that passes from mother to child during breastfeeding. Good bacteria are also passed along via vaginal births. Antibiotics, medications, and chlorine can kill off the body's natural flora and leave an undesirable imbalance of *Candida albicans* and other unhealthy bacteria, fungus or parasites. A diet high in simple carbohydrates, chemicals in the environment and in foods, and undetected allergies also degrade the natural flora. Supplementing with probiotics can help bring the population of healthy flora in your gut back into balance, and allow them to fulfill their true functionality.

Whey Protein

Protein is one of the major building blocks of your body. Eating high-quality protein with each meal repairs and rebuilds your body, stabilizes your blood sugar so you don't overeat, and helps stimulate a fat-burning hormone called glucagon. There are three primary categories (and some subcategories or fractions) of protein powder: caseinate, whey concentrate and whey isolate. Whey protein isolate is the higher-quality protein. It's easier to digest, is low in lactose or lactose-free, and, along with a good nutrition program, may enhance cell growth and repair. Whey even helps you maintain your healthy and ideal weight, as noted below:

• Whey controls your appetite. There's a compound in whey called glycomacropeptide that acts as a mild appetite suppressant.

- Whey balances blood sugar. It moderates the rate at which the energy of a balanced meal (containing carbohydrates, proteins and fats) enters your bloodstream. This keeps your blood sugar constant for longer, stopping cravings and excessive eating.

- Whey increases and supports muscle. The more muscle you have, the more calories your body burns.

When choosing whey protein at a health food store, it's important to select a high- quality product for optimum health benefits. By supplementing your diet with a high-quality, undenatured whey protein isolate, you can ensure your body's protein needs are being met, which will contribute to achieving and maintaining your ideal weight. Whey protein is a great product to use as a liquid meal in the form of a smoothie; you can visit **www.MindBodyFX.com** for a variety of delicious recipes. Whey is also great to use after a workout, as it goes to work immediately to enhance the rate of repair of your muscle tissue.

Note: If you're vegetarian, vegan or lactose intolerant, there are many other protein powders available for you. Look for one containing hemp, brown rice or split pea protein, or a combination of those ingredients.

Adrenal Support

Everyone experiences stress; it's how you deal with it that can become an issue. If you find your quality of life is compromised by your inability to handle stress, it's possible that your adrenal glands (responsible for the cascade of reactions that occur in your body during stress) have become exhausted and need support. Excess stress leads to obesity, and can also be a precursor to hypoglycemic symptoms, hormonal dysfunction (like PMS and menopausal symptoms), underactive thyroid, and underactive digestion.

There are specific and effective supplements that may be helpful in nourishing the adrenal glands to normalize and improve their function to more optimally support you in times of stress. Important nutrients for the adrenal glands are vitamin C (the urinary excretion of vitamin C is increased with stress), pantothenic acid (vitamin B5), vitamin B6, zinc, and magnesium. Essential fatty acids (EFAs) are essential for building hormones. Glandular, herbal or homeopathic support for the adrenal glands is also beneficial.

Thyroid Support

The thyroid gland regulates metabolism in every cell of your body, so a deficiency of thyroid hormone can affect virtually all body functions. Your thyroid produces the hormones T4 (thyroxine) and T3 (triiodothyronine). T4 is physiologically inactive, and must be converted to its active form, T3, before it can begin its work. Although some T3 is produced in the thyroid itself, most of the conversion occurs outside of the gland, using the enzyme deiodinase.

Supplements that contain nutrients to help to convert T4 to T3 may be effective in rebuilding the thyroid. Look for vitamins and minerals that are required to work together to manufacture thyroid hormones. Nutrients needed by the thyroid gland can be found either in supplements or foods containing B-complex vitamins, vitamin E, vitamin C, iodine, and select trace minerals and amino acids. Pituitary and thyroid glandulars are also very effective and are essentially a "custom meal" used temporarily for those particular glands.

Anti-Fungal Agents

Anti-fungal agents are used to reduce the overgrowth of *Candida albicans* (the yeast-like fungus that can get out of control in your body). What allows the *Candida albicans* to proliferate is a depressed and overwhelmed immune system, so restoring your immunity is essential. Everyone with candidiasis can acquire sensitivity to it; to bring *Candida* levels back to normal, you must first eliminate that sensitivity. This can be accomplished by taking a homeopathic remedy that includes ingesting a dilution of *Candida albicans* every day for two months while taking additional anti-fungal agents such as oil of oregano, garlic, grape seed extract, colloidal silver, caprylic acid and berberine-containing plants (goldenseal, barberry, and Oregon grape).

Essential Fatty Acids (EFAs)

EFAs are necessary fats that you can't make internally; they must be obtained through what you eat. There are two families of EFAs: omega-3 and omega-6. Omega-9 is necessary, yet is called non-essential, since your body can manufacture a modest amount on its own, provided other EFAs are present.

EFAs support the cardiovascular, reproductive, immune and nervous systems. Your body requires them for the manufacture and repair of cell membranes, enabling cells to obtain optimum nutrition and expel harmful waste products. A primary function of EFAs is the production of prostaglandins, which regulate functions such as heart rate, blood pressure, blood clotting, fertility and conception, and also play a role in immune function by regulating inflammation, decreasing histamine release, and encouraging the body to fight infection. EFAs are needed for proper growth in children, particularly for neural development and maturation of sensory systems.

While it's clear that EFAs are important to overall health, EFA deficiency is not uncommon in the U.S. An ideal intake ratio of omega-6 to omega-3 fatty acids is between 1:1 and 4:1, but most North Americans have ratios between 10:1 and 25:1. A link has been suggested between EFA deficiency and omega-6/omega-3 imbalance and health conditions such as heart attacks, cancer, insulin resistance, asthma, lupus, schizophrenia, depression, postpartum depression, accelerated aging, stroke, obesity, diabetes, arthritis, ADHD, and Alzheimer's disease.

Omega-3 (Linolenic Acid)

Omega-3s are used in the formation of cell walls, making them supple and flexible, and improving circulation and oxygen uptake with proper red blood cell flexibility and function. Omega-3 deficiencies have been linked to decreased memory and mental abilities, nerve tingling, poor vision, increased tendency to form blood clots, diminished immune function, increased triglycerides and "bad" cholesterol (LDL) concentrations, impaired membrane function, hypertension, irregular heartbeat, learning disorders, menopausal discomfort, and growth problems. Omega-3 is found in flaxseed oil (the highest omega-3 content of any food), flaxseeds, flaxseed meal, hempseed oil, hempseeds, walnuts, pumpkin seeds, Brazil nuts, butternuts, pecans, hazelnuts, sesame seeds, avocados, some dark leafy green vegetables (kale, spinach, purslane, mustard greens, collards, etc.), kiwis, wheat germ oil, salmon, mackerel, lake trout, sardines, anchovies, albacore tuna, and other foods in lower concentrations.

One tablespoon of flaxseed oil per day should provide the recommended daily adult portion of omega-3, although the time-released effects of consuming nuts and other omega-rich foods are being studied, to see if they're more beneficial than a once-daily oil intake. Flaxseed oil used for dietary supplementation should be kept in the refrigerator or freezer, and purchased from a supplier who refrigerates the liquid as well. Flaxseed oil loses its benefits and can become toxic if heated.

Omega-6 (Linoleic Acid)

Omega-6 is found in flaxseed oil, flaxseeds, flaxseed meal, hempseed oil, hempseeds, grape seed oil, pumpkin seeds, pine nuts, pistachio nuts, sunflower seeds (raw), olive oil, olives, borage oil, evening primrose oil, black currant seed oil, chestnut oil and chicken, among many others. Avoid refined and hydrogenated versions of these foods. Corn, safflower, sunflower, soybean, and cottonseed oils are also sources of omega-6, but are refined and may be nutrient-deficient as sold in stores.

Omega-6 can improve diabetes, rheumatoid arthritis, PMS, skin disorders (e.g., psoriasis and eczema), and aid in cancer treatment. Although most people obtain an excess of omega-6, it may not be converted into a usable form due to metabolic problems caused by diets rich in sugar, alcohol, or trans fats, as well as smoking, pollution, stress, aging, viral infections, and other illnesses like diabetes. It's best to eliminate these factors when possible, but some prefer to supplement with foods rich in omega-6 such as borage oil, black currant seed oil, nuts, eggs, whole grains, or evening primrose oil.

Green Powder (Greens)

It goes without saying that it's important to eat as many vegetables as possible. One way to increase your intake is to drink vegetables in the form of a green powder. There are many commercial powders on the market that contain highly concentrated nutrition that allow you to benefit from a multitude of vegetables, herbs, leaves, algae, seaweeds and grasses that you might otherwise find hard to include in your daily regime.

Your body easily absorbs the vitamins and minerals in green powder, making this an ideal supplement. Green powder contains a great supply of energy-creating nutrients, excellent for afternoon slumps. It also contains fiber, amino acids and chlorophyll, all essential for optimum health.

If you want what you do not have,
you must do what you have not done.
— **Unknown Author**

Getting Active!

The starting point of all achievement is desire.
Keep this constantly in mind. Strengthen your desire!
Weak desire brings weak results, just as a small
amount of fire makes a small amount of heat.

— Author Unknown

Many people blame their inability to achieve their ideal weight on a weak metabolism. It's important to understand what metabolism is, but also what it isn't. Metabolism is the chemical process through which your body converts food and other things into energy (calories). Whether you're eating, drinking, sleeping, cleaning or exercising, your body is constantly burning calories to keep you going.

Metabolism is affected by your particular body composition, which means the amount of muscle you have versus the amount of fat. Muscle uses more calories to maintain itself than fat, so people who are more muscular (and have a lower percentage of body fat) are said to have a higher metabolism than those who are less muscular. For example, let's say you have two people who are the exact same height and weight. One exercises on a regular basis with weights in addition to doing aerobic exercise, and has a low percentage of body fat. The other never exercises and has a higher percentage of body fat. The person who exercises will have a higher metabolism than the person who doesn't. What this means is that the first person's body will burn more calories to sustain itself than the second one.

People often ask how they can increase their metabolism, and it's really quite simple — so simple, in fact, that many people don't believe it. All you have to do is exercise and stop dieting. It's important to eat frequently, as your body requires fuel. Avoid skipping meals, enjoy healthy snacks between meals, and drink plenty of water.

You can increase your muscle mass by doing some type of resistance workout such as lifting weights. You can also decrease your level of body fat by doing some type of cardio exercise at least three days a week for as little as 20 minutes. By cardio exercise, I mean an activity that will increase your heart rate and keep it there for the duration of the exercise session (e.g., brisk walking, jogging, step aerobics, hi/low aerobics, biking, swimming).

Often individuals who never had a weight problem when they were young begin gaining as they age. After age 30, your body tends to lose its muscle tone. If your activity level and the number of calories you eat stay the same, you'll gain weight; your metabolism will have slowed down due to this loss of muscle tone, and your body will burn fewer of the calories you're taking in. You can forestall this natural tendency through exercise. If you work out with weights and do some type of cardio activity on a regular basis, you probably won't notice much of a change in your metabolism as you age.

Symptoms of slow metabolism include fatigue, feeling cold, dry skin, constipation, a slow pulse, low blood pressure, and, of course, weight gain. If you eat a very low-calorie diet, your body will slow its metabolism down in self-defense, holding onto whatever it can to survive. (Your body thinks it's starving.) If your diet has resulted in a loss of muscle and an increase in your percentage of body fat, then your metabolism has probably slowed down.

Metabolism and Genes

Genes do play a role in metabolism. Everyone has a different bone structure and body type. It's not realistic to think that everyone can look like a svelte beach beauty or a muscular body builder (without some serious effort). However, given your body type and genetic makeup, you can exercise (with weights and aerobically) to look the best you possibly can. Despite what you may believe, your genes won't prevent you from achieving your ideal weight.

Most experts agree that weight training and aerobic exercise increase metabolism during and after exercise. They disagree on how long after exercise your metabolism remains increased — that is, how long the excess post-exercise oxygen consumption lasts. Short-term effects on your metabolism depend mostly on the intensity of your workout, whether you're exercising aerobically or with weights (although it's far easier to raise your heart rate while exercising aerobically). When you exercise aerobically, focus on burning calories and working your cardiovascular system. Because it takes more calories to exercise, your metabolism speeds up during the activity.

When you're lifting weights or doing other resistance training, you can work out intensely and long enough to raise your heart rate, but most people choose to focus on the activity itself, which burns calories and also increases muscle strength, tone and endurance. This leads to longer-lasting effects on your metabolism. The combination of aerobic activity and weight training will result in a body that has more muscle and less fat, so the end result will be a higher metabolism.

Types Of Exercise

Walking

The simplest exercise of all, walking, can provide many health benefits: more energy, deeper and more satisfying sleep, stronger leg muscles, less knee pounding than running, lower body fat, a higher metabolic rate, and reduced stress. Taking walks on a daily basis can reduce your lifelong risks for heart disease, cancer, stroke, and high blood pressure, and may even slow the aging process.

While 30 to 60 minutes of walking per day is ideal, you can still benefit from increasing your walking by even a small amount. One thing that I highly recommend is using a pedometer, which counts the steps you actually take during the course of a day and allows you to measure your increases. Aim for a minimum pedometer reading of 10,000 steps every day.

One of the best things about walking is that it can be done anywhere; you don't have to make a trip to the gym or take extra time out of your day. Our lifestyles have changed from the past through dependence on vehicles, labor-saving devices, sedentary recreation, and a fast-paced lifestyle that leaves little room for dedicated physical activity…but we all still walk to some extent.

Due to family commitments or other issues, you may have a difficult time setting aside time for exercising, but you don't have to do that for walking. Significant health benefits can come from just 30 minutes of brisk walking on most days. Lunch and breaks are perfect times to get out for some fresh air and a walk around the block. You can also use the stairs instead of the elevator whenever possible, park your car farther away and walk an extra 10 minutes or so to your office, or use the bathroom on a different floor of your office building. Pick up the pace to burn more calories!

Yoga

If you've never tried yoga, you may be confused about what it is. Yoga is holding the body in a variety of poses that have been found to be beneficial for (isometric) strength, flexibility, balance, and concentration, and can be performed in conjunction with breathing exercises and meditation. It may release stress, as it's a calming activity. Yoga is extremely effective for the following:

Increasing flexibility. Yoga has positions that act on the various joints of your body, including those that are rarely exercised. Start by simply taking the time to stretch your arm, neck, and shoulder muscles when sitting in front of the computer. Try a few yoga stretches before bed; your back will thank you.

Increasing lubrication of the joints, ligaments and tendons. Likewise, the well-researched yoga positions exercise the different tendons and ligaments of the body. Surprisingly, it's been found that if you start a regular yoga regimen, your body, no matter how rigid you may have been before, can become remarkably flexible. Why? Seemingly unrelated "non-strenuous" yoga positions act on certain parts of the body in an interrelated manner, working in harmony to limber you up.

Massaging all organs of the body. Yoga is perhaps the only form of activity that massages all the internal glands and organs of the body in a thorough manner, including those — such as the prostate — that hardly get externally stimulated during your entire lifetime. Yoga acts in a healthful manner on the various body parts. This organ stimulation and massage benefits you by keeping away disease. It can also act as an early warning system for certain diseases or disorders.

Complete detoxification. By gently stretching muscles and joints as well as massaging various organs, yoga ensures the optimum blood supply to different parts of your body. This helps flush toxins from every area, which leads to benefits such as delayed aging, restored energy, and a renewed zest for life.

Excellent toning of the muscles. Muscles that have become flaccid or weak are stimulated repeatedly to shed excess flab and flaccidity through yoga. What yoga does is harmonize your mind and body. Through meditation, it helps your mind work in sync with your body. How often do you find that you're unable to perform your activities properly and in a satisfying manner because the confusions and conflicts in your mind weigh down heavily upon you? Moreover, yoga and meditation effectively counteract stress, which contributes to heart disease, affecting all parts of your physical, endocrinal, and emotional systems.

The meditative practices of yoga help in achieving an emotional balance by allowing you to temporarily detach from your surroundings, giving you a remarkable calmness and positive energy that has tremendous benefits on the physical health of your body. These are just some of the tangible benefits that can be achieved through yoga.

It's recommended that you engage in yoga twice a week to benefit from the mind/body connection. If you don't have the time to make it to a yoga class, you can always purchase a yoga DVD and practice yoga in the comfort of your own home first thing in the morning or after the kids go to bed. *The Complete MindBody FX Lifestyle Program* includes a bonus yoga DVD; you can learn more about this program at **www. MindBodyFX.com**.

Strength Training

Strength training usually takes the form of lifting weights, but it can be any activity that provides resistance for the muscles. There are numerous reasons and benefits for incorporating strength training into your workout:

Increased metabolic rate. Strength training increases your body's long-term metabolic rate, causing it to burn more calories throughout the day.

Increased and restored bone density. Inactivity and aging can lead to a decrease in bone density and brittleness. Studies have clearly proven that consistent strength training can increase bone density and prevent osteoporosis.

Increased lean muscle mass and muscle strength, power, and stamina. Everyone can benefit from being stronger. You can work harder, play more, work out longer, and feel more alive.

Injury prevention. Strengthening muscles and joints can prevent a wide variety of injuries.

Improved balance, flexibility, mobility and stability. Stronger and more resilient muscles improve your balance, which means more comfortable living and fewer falls or accidents.

Decreased risk of coronary disease. Participation in a consistent strength-training program has a wide variety of affiliated health benefits, including decreasing cholesterol and lowering blood pressure.

Improved rehabilitation and recovery. One of the best ways to heal many types of injuries is to strengthen the muscles surrounding the injured area. The stronger your muscles, the quicker the healing process.

Enhanced performance in sports or exercise. No matter what your favorite sport or physical activity might be, with the proper strength training program, your performance can unquestionably be improved, and in some cases dramatically so.

Aging gracefully. There may be no more important reason to making strength training a consistent part of your life than to ensure you age gracefully. Physical activity keeps you alive and vibrant. Strength training ensures that you're strong enough to participate in aerobic activities, outdoor recreation, sexual activity and sports. Strong seniors fall down less often, and are less apt to be injured if they do. Their stronger bodies are more resilient, and if they're injured, they heal more quickly.

Feeling better and looking better. Stronger muscles and joints can have a dramatic impact on posture. Lean, toned muscles can also make you feel better about your appearance. This all leads to improved self-esteem and increased self-confidence.

Cardio Training

Cardio training includes walking, jogging, swimming, or any type of activity that works numerous major muscle groups and gets your heart pumping harder for the duration of the exercise. You can start by walking, riding a stationary bike, getting on a treadmill or elliptical trainer, using a stair-stepping machine, or doing aerobics. Cardio should be incorporated into your workout regime at least three times a week.

Once your fitness level begins to improve, you'll need to increase the intensity of your cardio training to get past fitness and weight-reduction plateaus. You can do this by incorporating high-intensity intervals into your existing cardio program. If you walk or bike at a fairly consistent pace for 30 minutes, try speeding it up for one minute every few minutes. If you use an aerobics video, you can up the intensity by watching one of the more advanced participants and trying to keep up with that person for 30 to 60 seconds at a time. As you become more fit, you can try various combinations.

Once your fitness level increases, you can reduce the walking time and have more frequent running intervals. (Interval training is one of the most effective methods for fat release, as it increases your levels of growth hormone, which is responsible for increasing fat breakdown, anti-aging, immune system stimulation, and increasing muscle repair and growth of all the internal organs except the brain.) The key is to constantly challenge your body so you release fat and reduce weight more rapidly. Another benefit of incorporating intervals into your cardio program is that it alleviates boredom. Regular cardio training also helps prevent a variety of medical conditions, including heart attack, diabetes, high blood pressure, high cholesterol, and obesity... and you can expect to have more energy, higher endurance, and less stress, as well as better sleep, more calories burned, and an easier time achieving your ideal weight!

Exercise And Emotions

More Americans than ever are joining their local gym or health club. The problem is this isn't enough. You have to actually go. There are many excuses not to exercise, but here I'd like to concentrate on emotions. If you're like many adults, you feel over-committed, over-scheduled, and over-stressed, and the mere thought of rearranging your life to squeeze in something else feels overwhelming.

So...don't. That is, don't just rearrange your schedule; change your life. Throughout this book, I've emphasized the role the power of the mind plays in your life. By now you know that the first step down the path toward achieving your goals — and your ideal weight — is preparing your mind. It's time to stop thinking about what you don't want or think you can't do and replace those thoughts with what you do want and what you can do. This is the perfect time to re-evaluate everything in your life, from how you eat to how you relax. Revisit your priorities now that you've adopted your new, positive mindset, and many of those time and energy commitments you thought would make regular exercise impossible may simply fall by the wayside. You shouldn't feel overwhelmed; you should feel in control.

The good news is that regular exercise can actually help you think positively. As with everything else worth achieving, however, that won't happen overnight. When you begin your new routine, whatever it may be — running, aerobics, swimming, cardio-kickboxing, spinning, circuit training — you'll go through some changes. When you first hit the gym or the trail, you'll feel exhilarated and resolute. No matter how much exercise you actually manage that first day, when you hit the shower, you'll feel pretty darn proud of yourself, and rightly so. But if you aren't used to doing anything physical, after a few hours and especially when you get up the next morning, you'll probably feel exhausted, with aches and pains in muscles that haven't been worked in ages. You may feel that you have barely enough energy to get through the regular parts of your day, let alone exercise. This is temporary! Don't let your body's minor complaints sway your mind's determination to change.

No matter how difficult it may be to lace up those running shoes or get on that stair-step machine, push away those thoughts of "This is too hard" and "I'll never be able to do this." Here's one way to avoid some of that almost-inevitable disillusionment: When you plan your new exercise program, don't design it for your 20-year-old self (unless, of course, you're 20), especially if you've lived a largely sedentary life. Challenge yourself, but don't set goals so unrealistic that you're guaranteed to fail.

Once you make it past the first few days, the first few weeks, and the first few months, you'll notice a strange phenomenon: adding a regular regimen of aerobic activity gives you more energy, not less. That's because your metabolism changes. When you're largely sedentary, your heart pumps oxygen-rich blood to every part of your body at a relatively slow and steady rate. When you exercise enough to raise your heart rate, your blood flows faster, reaching and rejuvenating all your body's cells, and carrying blood to and from your organs, for example, your liver, which (among other things) removes trace toxins and waste elements. Regular exercise also builds up muscle mass, a far more active and efficient metabolizer than love handles and spare tires.

Speaking of energy, don't fall victim to what Dr. Judith Orloff (Positive Energy, Harmony Books) calls "energy vampires." She identifies four types: the constant victim, who recounts every major trauma and minor slight; the charmer, who must be in the spotlight at all times; the drama queen (or king), for whom life is always either incredibly wonderful or a terrible tragedy; and the blamer, whose specialty is making others feel guilty.

These "vampires" are people who, rather than boosting our spirits and energies, sap it all away, leaving us tired and distressed. The energy vampires you may meet (and should avoid!) as you introduce your new fitness program are, in Orloff's parlance, these:

- Victims will stop you during your workout to list all the diseases and conditions that keep them from being able to do whatever it is you're trying to do.

- Charmers will teach aerobics or play racquetball with such boundless energy and enthusiasm that you'll feel inadequate and discouraged.

- Drama queens will get you all excited about a new class and then, when you sign up, tell you they heard someone died in that class.

- Blamers will complain that now that you're exercising, you never spend any time with them going to lunch or the movies, or just hanging out.

These people will sabotage you if you let them! Don't let the energy vampires' emotions dampen yours.

Exercising can actually improve your mood, although in the beginning, you may not notice it, or you may even experience the opposite. That's normal. After all, the results of all your exertions are not immediately obvious.

Some people, particularly those already prone to skin problems, may experience some acne breakouts. The prevention and remedy for that is simple: shower with soap as soon as possible after you work up a sweat. Acne may very well improve once the toxins in your body have had a chance to be eliminated and your adrenal system is functioning correctly.

During and for a while after strenuous exercise, you may feel a significant improvement in your mood. This comes from anandamides (a natural cannabinoid) and endorphins (chemicals released by the pituitary and hypothalamus glands) that act as natural painkillers and mood boosters. A study done at Duke University Medical Center showed that engaging in a regular exercise program was as effective in treating mild depression as one of the more popular antidepressants. This "high" can actually help you stick to your routine, as many people become addicted — psychologically, at least.

The difference between try and triumph is just a little umph!

— Marvin Phillips

Finding Support

Obstacles are what we see when we take our eyes off the goal.

— **Rita Davenport**

It's very hard, if not impossible, to try to make life changes by yourself. You don't live in a void; you interact with friends, family and coworkers constantly, and these individuals can be a wonderful source of support. Unfortunately, they can also be less than helpful at times and even add to the stress you feel when embarking on a new healthy lifestyle.

I've put together some tips to help you get the most out of your existing support system and some ideas for adding more support from other sources. After all, we all need a little help now and then. When you become truly committed to your new healthy lifestyle, it's perfectly reasonable, and often essential, to ask your loved ones to become key participants with you.

Tips For Getting the Best Support From Family and Friends

1. **Ask for encouragement.** Often you embark on a new exercise regime or weight reduction plan and expect the world to cheer automatically. This doesn't always happen. Let your family and friends know what you're up to, and that you'd like a little boost of encouragement every now and then. Let them know how much you appreciate their support when they help keep you motivated.

2. **Make one area of your house a designated eating zone** — and the rest off limits for food. This area will probably be the kitchen and/or dining room for most families. Ask everyone's help; banish snacking in front of the TV or in bedrooms. It's very hard to resist temptation while the person next to you munches buttery popcorn.

3. **Put a chart or progress report in plain view for all to see and ask others to celebrate milestones with you (in non-food celebrations).** Your celebrations can include going to see a movie (bringing your own snacks), getting a manicure or massage, or buying yourself something special. Frequently people have the tendency to keep their weight information private, but if everyone sees your progress, everyone can encourage you...and they may even be inspired to take charge of their own health and eating habits.

4. **Meet with your family or friends and talk about the guidelines of your new program.** Discuss how others can help you meet your goals and pinpoint problem areas before they have a chance to negatively affect your plan. For example, if you frequently have lunch with friends, suggest locations with healthy menu choices.

5. **Clean out the pantry and label one shelf as yours.** Place all your healthy items and snacks on your shelf. When you're tempted to reach for anything in the pantry, your shelf will be right there filled with treats that won't blow your goals. Either ban junk food entirely or insist that it be stored elsewhere.

6. **Learn to share!** Tell others about your successes. When you pass a particular milestone, let others see how enthusiastic and happy you are to be accomplishing your goals. By sharing in your joy, people will see how important this is to you and will therefore be even more likely to support you.

7. **Potluck passion.** Make family get-togethers and dinners healthier by preparing entrees or side dishes that are in keeping with your new eating plan. That way, you'll always have something good to eat and you'll allow others to have a taste...and maybe even join you.

8. **Plan, plan, plan.** There will often be those in the family who need some convincing that healthy food tastes good. If you have small children or a resistant spouse, be sure to plan meals well in advance so you don't munch from their food choices just because it's quick and easy. Keep track of recipes you like that fit with your new way of eating. Eventually, you'll have your own great cookbook of healthy and delicious tasting meals, so you don't fall back to your old way of eating.

Why Won't They Help?

Anyone who's set out on a new healthy lifestyle has encountered a friend or family member who's been less than helpful. It's important to be prepared for the frustrating interference of loved ones who don't approve of or understand your desire to reduce your weight to look and feel better about yourself. Most of us will at some point have someone in our lives who will innocently — or knowingly — try to sabotage our efforts. Usually these types of people have ulterior motives for their desire to keep things as they are, and often it stems from their own insecurities.

Sometimes it all comes down to one ugly four-letter word: fear. Do your friends or family feel the new, svelte you will move on to things they don't enjoy? Perhaps fellow singletons fear that your social life may improve and you'll be dating instead of socializing with them. Maybe your healthier ways are making your friends feel guilty about their own less-than-perfect eating habits. Or worse, maybe you make them feel better about their own weight issues because they're overweight, too, and you may be heavier than they are, so next to you they look and feel thinner.

Many of our social activities revolve around food...dinner with friends, movies with popcorn and soda, Happy Hour with the gang, or family gatherings. When you change the way you eat, the way you relate to your friends and family (with food) changes, too. To get the "old you" back, some may try to push food on you or try to entice you into joining them in their couch potato existence. A key in preventing or solving this situation is communication. Make it clear from the onset that you're serious about releasing weight and that you need their help to make it happen.

If you feel unsupported by those who you think should be your biggest cheerleaders, you'll probably find yourself searching for the reasons why — and there isn't an easy answer. Anyone who truly loves you will want what's best for you and your health. If you think you've reached an unhealthy weight and you finally feel ready to change, reducing those excess pounds safely and steadily should become a priority for everyone around you. Eventually, most of the people in your life will see that what you're doing is a good thing — even if it does slightly alter your social life or family functions. Do your best to get those around you to not only encourage you, but to jump on the bandwagon with you toward healthier living...then everyone benefits.

If you find you don't get the support you need at home, or if you're new to an area and don't have your usual support system, there are other places to turn. Studies have shown that people who use online support are far more likely to succeed in their weight and health goals than those who try to go it alone. Many websites offer forums for those who are going through similar issues to connect and chat; there are always numerous supportive community members ready to talk about healthy eating, share tips on motivation, and discuss whatever else may be on your mind, and you can access this support system any time and from anywhere.

Even if you find great support with an online community, sometimes nothing can replace the connection with real people on a personal level. There are plenty of face-to-face support groups you can join if you find online communities a little impersonal. I've provided a few examples below.

- Many community health centers, senior centers, community colleges, and universities offer programs focused on health and well-being. Some will allow access to medical, nutritional or fitness specialists for free or a nominal fee.

- Medical facilities often offer special programs to help with weight issues — especially if you have additional risk factors such as diabetes or high blood pressure. While these wellness programs often cost a bit more, many insurance companies will help offset your investment.

- Join a walking club. If you can't find one in your area, then create one. Studies show that overweight people tend to spend most of their time with other overweight people. Likewise, physically fit people spend their time with other physically fit people. Join a group of physically fit people and you'll begin to think like them, which will bring about positive results in both your mind and body!

- Fitness centers often have nutritionists on staff who can get you involved in their programs and meetings. Don't think you have to spend a lot of money. Often the local YMCA will offer free programs you can join.

- Be a leader. Why not form your own MindBody FX support group with family, friends and co-workers? The more people around you who are working toward the same goal, the easier it will be for you! There's more information about how to create your own support group available at **www.MindBodyFX.com**.

Releasing weight doesn't have to mean losing your old friends, and it can even mean making new ones. You can team up with someone and set a date to exercise together. When you make an appointment to workout, you're far more likely to actually show up and do it. Research shows that having a buddy can help you stick to your healthy eating habits, too. A buddy can give you determination when temptation strikes and is only a phone call away. One of my clients and her out-of- town siblings started emailing each other to report the amount of time they spent exercising or walking each day. They each agreed to commit to at least six hours a week, and nicknamed themselves "skinny minnies." This teamwork has really helped to keep them committed to their goals; it makes them to think twice about sleeping past the alarm in the morning or making an excuse not to go to the gym.

One of the best ways to choose the right person to be your MindBody FX buddy is to identify your own problem areas. For example, if you tend to snack late at night, find another late-night snacker with whom you can talk on the phone rather than reaching for that ice cream or chocolate. If the vending machine at work is your weakness, buddy up with a co-worker who also fights the mid-afternoon munchies, and share a walk around the block instead.

The best part about finding another person to team up with is that it's likely your relationship will eventually be about more than eating healthy or exercising together. It could be the start of a beautiful friendship that's positive and nurturing.

Get A Life Or Health Coach

One alternative that many people opt for these days is hiring a life coach to help them improve their lives or personal performance in all sorts of areas, such as stress management, business, weight reduction, personal relationships, and dozens more. These professionals can help you gain self-knowledge, create more effective goals, and work with you to create a plan and framework that you'll use to go about accomplishing those goals. One of the biggest functions a life coach can provide is assistance with any underlying issues that might be preventing you from succeeding. If you've tried many health regimes in the past and haven't found success, this is a great option.

Ten Ways A Life Or Health Coach Can Help You

Life coaches can provide certain benefits you can't experience when embarking on the journey alone. Here are 10 reasons a life coach may be right for you:

1. **Motivation.** One of the main benefits of having a life coach is to receive additional motivation to stick with a consistent program. A life coach can provide structure and accountability and help you develop a lifestyle that encourages health.

2. **Individualized programs.** If you have any chronic health conditions, injuries, or health goals, a life coach can work with you and your healthcare provider to plan a safe, efficient program that takes your "full picture" into account and enables you to reach your goals. A life coach can also help you determine what goals need to be adjusted, depending on those considerations.

3. **Efficiency.** A life coach helps you focus and maintain your purpose. This makes it much easier to stay on target and not waste time starting and stopping your health program.

4. **Improved mental skills.** Once you're able to understand the belief systems that have hindered you in the past, a life coach can encourage new thoughts and affirmations that soon become part of your thought process. This allows you to replace old beliefs with new, positive beliefs about yourself.

5. **Starting points.** If you're an absolute beginner, a life coach can show you tried-and-true methods to achieve your purpose and vision, offering you simple steps to start accomplishing goals that are in line them.

6. **Break through plateaus.** Even if you feel you're in relatively good health, a life coach can help you break out of your routine and stretch your boundaries, infusing you with new energy, ideas, and passion for life that you may have forgotten over time.

7. **A plan for going it alone.** If you ultimately want to learn all the facets of maintaining your new lifestyle, a life coach can set you on the journey to good health for the rest of your life. Once you understand your own basic motivations and weaknesses, your coach can provide you the tools you'll need to take it from there if you choose.

8. **Safe workouts.** A life coach may also recommend a personal trainer who can watch your form while you exercise and provide objective feedback about your limits and strengths. Exercise isn't a one-size-fits-all proposition. There may be certain physical skills you don't have, aren't ready for yet, or your body doesn't respond to as well. Most of us tend to ignore some of the subtle signals our body provides; we either push through pain or give up too soon. By directing you toward physical activities that you like and that work for you, a life coach can keep your interest high and improve your chances for success.

9. **Convenience.** Many life coaches will accommodate your schedule. This is the number-one reason most people cite for hiring one. You're busy, and often gyms and colleges don't offer classes or help when it fits your schedule.

10. **Your ideal weight.** As a coach myself, I specialize in helping people achieve their ideal weight. There's a good reason that so many people want the help of a coach. I can keep people on track and help them realize their goals and achieve life-long results. So many of the people I talk with have tried just about everything out there and not met with success in the long term. Since my approach is to first understand how each person thinks and how that's affecting their outcomes, my clients are able to achieve the long-term success that's previously eluded them. A healthy lifestyle is not a short-term or one-shot endeavor; it's an ongoing way to live that can bring you tremendous rewards.

Finding Balance

Balance means that you have a sense that all the parts of your life form a harmonious whole. Balance is different for everyone, and even different for you at various stages of your life. You may work long hours, but if that produces your desired rewards and allows you enough time to enjoy some leisure pursuits while maintaining your health goals, you're likely to feel balanced and stable.

When you're off-balance, on the other hand, the smallest thing, such as an unexpected deadline, can send you over the edge. Indeed, when things get overwhelming, you lose your balance. This can result in a backslide into old habits: emotional eating, lack of exercise, and a reluctance to try something new.

Balance can be a tricky thing to hold onto in your life, as it always seems to be a moving target. The key to balance is to be in control of yourself and your goals, to keep moving in a forward direction, and to accept that sometimes you need to take a backward or sideways step to maintain your momentum.

Your sense of balance changes with your life priorities, as the excitement of new goals fades a little and as you become more comfortable with who you are. When you're a young adult, you may be prepared to put a great deal of energy into your work and social life because it may be very important to you to prove yourself, to earn the money you want, and to have fun — while you hardly give your health a second thought. When you reach your 40s and beyond, you may be ready to look past many of your material goals and find you want to spend more time rediscovering yourself and trying out new things. You may also realize that you're given only one body and that failing to take care of it will likely shorten your lifespan, and definitely decrease your quality of life!

I've put together the following list of ways you can step back from the chaos and stress of everyday life and create balance in your day and life.

Opportunities For Balance

- Take 10 minutes and envision what you want to achieve. Enjoy the simple act of seeing, hearing and living your ideal future. Relax and enjoy the moment.

- Understand and remind yourself each day of all you have to be thankful for. A grateful heart allows positive feelings to flow through your body. Take time during each day to list several things you're grateful for, beginning first thing in the morning by saying who and what you're grateful for out loud.

- Balance your own needs and goals with random acts of kindness. Do one thing each day to improve someone else's life. Let someone with only a few groceries go ahead of you, hold a door open or smile at a stranger.

- Collect wise quotes. Listen and read the words of those who've been through circumstances like yours and understand their message of hope. Read affirmations to yourself every single day. Post them in sight so you can easily see them in times of stress.

- Allow yourself time for reflection. Some days it seems you go all day without a break. Take a few minutes and allow your mind to reflect on the events of the day.

- Take a few deep breaths and slow down for just a few minutes — in traffic, in line at the store, wherever you are.

- Take a walk. You probably spend more time indoors than you realize. Allow yourself a few minutes each day to commune with nature. Notice the change of seasons and allow your heart to soar.

- Be kind to yourself. Forgive any faltering from your plan and keep pushing onward.

To receive a Free Special Report called Tips and Tools for Implementing a Healthier Lifestyle go to **www.mindbodyfx.com/ specialreport1**.

Every time you are tempted to react in the same old way,
ask if you want to be a prisoner of the past or a pioneer of the future.
—Deepak Chopra

Beginning Your New Life

With the past, I have nothing to do;
nor with the future. I live now.

— **Ralph Waldo Emerson**

As you've read this book, you'll have noticed how large a portion of it is spent on preparing your mind to meet your health goals. If you've been involved in weight loss or fitness programs in the past, you know how hard it is to start again and face the risk of failure. I'm sure that you experience many fears and frustrations when trying to reduce weight...but I want you to know that this time it will be different. Why? Because you now believe you can do it and you can see the end result in your mind.

We've discussed how obsessed we are as a population with quick fixes and shortcuts; this is not one of them. This is a lifestyle change, not a one-shot deal. You won't go back to being one of those people who takes good health for granted and continues on the weight loss/gain rollercoaster ride. The fact that you're searching for answers is the key to finding those solutions.

The purpose of this final chapter is to summarize all that's been covered in this book, so you know where to start and what steps you need to take to ensure that you achieve your goal of attaining your ideal weight.

Write Down Your Goal

Write down what your goal is, and see it in your mind's eye. Feel it in your heart and want it with all your might. Find a photo of yourself at your ideal weight, even if you have to cut out a picture from a magazine and paste your smiling face on it. Post it on your fridge or bathroom mirror; inside the cover of this book or in your journal; or at your desk. When you set your goal, really think about it. Remember a goal that's lightly set will be abandoned at the first obstacle. Choose your own goal; others may try to persuade you to follow their vision, but you must pursue your own. You need to own your goal, so be firm about this.

Visualize

Take a look around you. Everything you see was once a thought in someone's mind. Disneyland, the light bulb, the telephone, the car, the airplane — they all started as a small seed of thought in the mind of some brave soul who dared to imagine. Just as everything that's been created started with the thought in someone's mind, so can your ideal weight.

Be sure to take the time for yourself each day to visualize your ideal weight. As you visualize what you want and create the belief within your subconscious mind, the Law of Attraction will assist your efforts by clearing the path and allowing you to find those who can help you. This is not to say your path will be without obstacles. If you've struggled with emotional eating in the past, it will occasionally rear its ugly head. As you become more aware of your own triggers, you'll be able to abandon this type of eating, along with any "diet victim" excuses you may have used to this point. You have the ability to take control and get what you want. Now use that power to your benefit! As you begin new healthy habits, the daily affirmations you say to yourself will help you through the rough spots.

Follow The Mindbody FX Nutrition Plan

Focus on healthy eating and become aware of what you put in your mouth and why. Make a copy of the nutrition plan provided in this book and carry it with you. Make several copies: one for your fridge, one for your wallet and even one for your support person.

Follow and remember the **Daily Eating Habit Guidelines**:

1. Eat three to six meals and snacks or mini-meals throughout the day.
2. Eat breakfast soon after waking.
3. Include sources of whole foods carbohydrates, proteins and fats with each meal or snack.
4. Include vegetables or fruit with each meal.
5. Eat a rainbow of produce.
6. Drink adequate water each and every day.
7. Eat until you are 80% full.
8. Live by the 80/20 rule.

Plan your week's menu in advance and prepare your shopping list to carry with you to the grocery store. Make a point of visiting health food stores and farmers markets, where you'll find great quality, fresh whole foods. Eat organic whenever possible. By ridding your body of toxins, you'll be doing an internal cleansing, and you'll soon feel better than you have in years, or even decades! This newfound energy will get you moving off the couch and make you want to start moving and working your muscles. You may find yourself at ballroom dance lessons or wanting to run a marathon. Whatever it is, it will be an excellent boost not only for you, but also for those around you. Life is just beginning!

Drink Plenty of Water

I need to stress again how important it is to drink plenty of water — specifically alkaline water (refer to the section on water for more about alkalinity). Not only is it life giving, it hydrates every cell, allowing your body to function at its highest efficiency. Write down how much water you're currently drinking and what your target is, and then write out your plan and commitment to drinking the right amount of water each day.

Set a schedule to get yourself to the ideal level, noting it in your PDA or day planner. If you currently drink two glasses of water a day, increase it gradually. Aim for three tomorrow, then four a few days later, and so on, until you're naturally drinking a minimum of eight to 10 glasses a day.

The benefits of drinking water are undeniable. You'll have more energy, look younger, and feel more vibrant than you have in years. Your skin will radiate its gratitude.

Use Nutritional Supplements

Daily supplements are also important, and some of the more important ones have been outlined for you in this book. There may be others you want to add that you feel will help your particular situation. I've offered only a few of the most important ones, so don't hesitate to add to my list if you feel something additional will benefit you. Remember one thing, though: there's no magic pill, and these supplements should be taken only as a healthy part of your MindBody FX Lifestyle and not as the key ingredient in your nutrition plan. Nothing comes close to the complete nutritional value of fresh food as nature intended.

Surround Yourself With Support

I also want to reiterate how important it is to get the support you need. Your success is too important to attempt to go it alone. Get everyone you know on your side and rooting for you! If you need to, give your kids a dollar for every time they stop you from putting your hand in their chip bag, ordering French fries, or popping open a cold beer. Get a coach or join a group coaching program to gain support and accountability. If you have someone to keep you accountable, you'll be more likely to complete a task. Do whatever you feel is necessary to stack the odds in your favor to achieve your ultimate success, even creating your own support group to get the additional encouragement you need. For more information on creating your own MindBody FX Support Group, go to **www.MindBodyFX.com**.

Track Your Progress

Keep a written log of how you're doing each day. This way, you have a record of how far you've come, so you can praise yourself for a job well done. Record everything you've eaten (both the healthy and the not so healthy). How much water or other beverages have you consumed? How much activity have you enjoyed? How are you feeling emotionally and physically? How are you sleeping? Did you wake up feeling fantastic and ready to go, or did you want to hide under the covers when the alarm went off? On a scale of 1 to 10, how were your energy levels? What supplements did you take? What positive affirmations did you focus on? When you begin and then once a month, get out a measuring tape and record your measurements and if you choose to weigh yourself, only do so once a month as well. Keep track of how you feel after meals and after eating certain foods. Eliminate those foods that don't make you to feel well. You can buy a blank journal to record all of this or get the MindBody FX Journal.

Focus on Repetition

Repetition and practice are the keys to learning a new skill. Read this book several times, perhaps a chapter a night. After a couple of weeks, read it again. Review your goal and your motivation to achieve it regularly. Never change your actual goal, only the steps required to achieve it if something isn't working for you.

Begin Your Journey

Since this is the last chapter, I'd like to get you started on your path to success. The first thing I'm going to ask you to do is take a few minutes and answer some questions about your health and wellness goals. These are designed to make you really think about what you want. They will also uncover some truths about your relationship with food and exercise. Please write your answers in the spaces provided, or in your journal. This will provide a record of where you started and what your mindset was when you embarked on this journey to your ideal weight.

MY HEALTH AND WELLNESS GOALS

1. How have my feelings about my health and weight changed over the years?

   _____

   _____

   _____

2. **What's really important to me right now about my health and weight?** List as many things as you can think of (e.g., getting in shape, reducing my weight, having more energy, etc.).

   _____

   _____

   _____

3. What is my number one health and wellness goal right now?

   _____

   _____

   _____

4. **How has my definition of good health changed over the years?** Good health at one time in your life may have meant having the stamina to burn the candle at both ends. Now, good health may mean giving your body rest, and taking care of your mental and emotional well-being through gentle exercise and meditation.

   _____

   _____

   _____

5. **How much time do I want to allocate to my health and well-being?** Reaching and maintaining overall good health takes time

and effort. Consider whether you want to devote a regular daily time slot to your health goals or if a weekly commitment is better.

_____

_____

_____

6. **How do I want to feel when I think about my health?** You can translate this desire into a positive affirmation such as, "I feel strong, energetic and full of vitality every day!"

_____

_____

_____

7. **What do I want for my future health and well-being?** Perhaps you want to reduce your weight by 20 pounds or run a marathon, or simply be disease-free and enjoy life.

_____

_____

_____

This short questionnaire will give you a good idea of your starting point. Your body deserves respect and loving care. A great starting point for holistic health (the concept that physical, mental, and emotional health are all connected and have an impact on each other) is getting used to being comfortable in your own skin and changing the way you think and feel about your body. Replace the negative thoughts about your body that pop into your head with positive ones. Succeeding in health and overall well-being usually works best when you focus on what's already working and figure out how to do more of that, or when you enhance what you already have and add great new habits to it.

Hereditary and environmental factors that affect your health are not always within your full control. No matter what your genetic makeup is, however, and no matter what kind of air you have to breathe, you can still actively control and change your diet and the exercise you get. Diet and exercise can make a massive difference in how healthy you are now and will remain throughout your life.

Don't Forget Exercise

If you're already fairly healthy, you may just want to take your fitness to the next level. If this is your health goal, then you need to shift into a higher gear and commit to a sustained program that allows you to participate in your chosen exercise for 30 to 60 minutes for at least four out of seven days each week to achieve a real change in your fitness level. Get out there and do it; your body will thank you.

Increased fitness gives you more energy on a daily basis, strengthens bones and joints, helps you become more toned, makes you look and feel younger, reduces stress, allows you to play games with your children, improves your posture, and most importantly, increases your self-esteem. These benefits are all within your grasp through a well-chosen fitness strategy. If you want to achieve all these benefits, keep the following suggestions in mind:

- Choose a number of different forms of exercise. Start by listing the ones you know you'll enjoy and then list the ones you'd like to try. Choose at least one from each list.

- Set realistic long-term goals, but always stretch a bit beyond. Begin by checking off the exercises you know you'll do for at least 20 minutes a day.

- Schedule exercise into your PDA with a reminder alarm, or write it on the calendar on your fridge.

- Accept that you need to spend some of your time pursuing your health goals, perhaps at the expense of other activities.

- Choose the form of exercise that works for you and also inspires and motivates you to keep at it through the days, weeks, and months to come.

SET YOUR OWN EXERCISE AND FITNESS GOALS

Fitness means different things to different people. Only by examining your preconceived ideas can you set goals that are in keeping with your overall health goals. Take a few moments and think about these questions.

1. **What does "fitness" mean to you?** It could mean running a mile in less than five minutes, walking around the block or up a flight of stairs without getting winded, or participating in a marathon.

    _____

    _____

    _____

    _____

2. **What environment do you enjoy when you're participating in physical activity?** For some this would be the outdoors, for others a gym, and still others prefer team sports. List your preferences.

    _____

    _____

    _____

    _____

3. **How fit were you when you were young?** Were you a star player on the team or a spectator? This will determine your level of understanding of how your body responds to activity and how much you'll be able to handle.

    _____

    _____

    _____

    _____

4. **What environment do you work in and what opportunities does it offer for additional fitness?** Does your building have

stairs? Do you lift objects frequently? Is there a company sports team you can join? Can you park farther away from the entrance?

_____

_____

_____

_____

5. **What steps can you take to incorporate fitness into your everyday life?** Do you walk to neighborhood stores and shops? Can you park farther away when shopping? Can you walk up and down stairs in your home while on the phone? Think of ways to be active and list them.

_____

_____

_____

_____

For a Free Checklist to keep you on track with your goal of achieving your ideal weight go to **www.mindbodyfx.com/checklist**.

Whether your exercise of choice is strapping on a pedometer and setting off on a walk or practicing yoga, I encourage you to occasionally change your routine to keep things interesting. Don't forget that physical activity has a direct and positive impact on your mental well-being. It can also be very helpful in managing your emotions.

Do you feel comfortable expressing your emotions, or do you bottle things up only to find they explode at just the wrong moment? Do you notice what your emotions are all the time, or do you find you sometimes feel upset but can't really put your finger on why? Often when your physical well-being is out of sync, your emotions are as well. This can result in anger, emotional tears and even panic. These emotions have a physical effect on your body that can be released through regular, healthy exercise. Exercise gives your mind a chance to work through any emotional issues, and it also releases endorphins, a natural chemical from the pituitary gland that spreads a feeling of calm and happiness through your body.

Recall times when you've experienced various emotions and describe what the physical feeling is for you. Perhaps "joy" or "pride" brings on a warm sensation to the back of your throat, or thinking of the word "motivation" causes a pleasant tension in your abdomen. Notice the similarities and differences between each positive emotion. Now think about the negative emotions you experience. Maybe "anger" causes your shoulders to tense while "lonely" gives you an empty feeling in your stomach.

A positive thought isn't just an idea; it has a positive physical effect…and regular exercise can increase that effect. Armed with this awareness, you can now watch yourself as you go about your day and notice your feelings. When someone cuts you off in traffic, how do you feel? Angry? Frustrated? Rejected? You might be surprised at the real emotion behind the trigger and that it can change depending on the mood you're in to begin with. By maintaining a positive outlook, it's less likely that a negative event will ruin your day or steer you off course from achieving your goal weight.

You can make a big impact on your emotional well-being by simply noticing the things that make you feel good and going out of your way to make them part of your life. Those mornings when you wake up full of enthusiasm for no particular reason don't come out of thin air. Your mind takes what you give it, and if you're supplying positive thoughts while feeding your body healthy food and exercising regularly, then of course you'll wake up feeling great most of the time! That's a welcome and gratifying way to start your day.

Your eventual success will depend on your level of mental resilience and how quickly you can bounce back from setbacks. If you feel you're wobbling on the edge, about to slide into old habits due to external pressures and feeling out of control, you're not alone. Many people who seem to be very healthy and fit have at some time or another suffered from weight gain and couch potato syndrome. Recently, a friend of mine went hiking in the snow. The next day her legs were extremely sore, but her husband wanted to go hiking again. Even though it was snowing hard, they headed out. Before long, she started complaining about how sore her legs were and swearing that she didn't think she could continue. All she could think of was how good it would feel to get back home and put her feet up. Her husband was the support she needed that day. He kept her focused on the moment, reminded her how toned her legs were going to be, and described the nice bath she could take when she finished the hike. She persisted through the discomfort. She did reward herself with a hot bubble bath later that night, but what felt even better was her feeling of accomplishment!

Developing mental resilience begins with some basic strategies that can help you grow stronger:

- Talk to someone who can help you when you experience setbacks, like a life coach.

- Have a friend who can be there for you. You don't get an award for bravery for going it alone. Enlist the advice of a doctor or trained counselor if volatile emotions become persistent and overwhelming.

- Keep focused on your priorities. You may need to practice saying "no" from time to time. When you feel less mentally resilient, you may try to please people more, or go in the other direction and get angry at the demands they place on you. Knowing your goals and reminding yourself of them often can be the sanity check you require to assert your needs.

- Schedule a regular activity that builds your mental and emotional muscles. Take note of activities that leave you with a sense of peace and perspective and give them priority in your life. This may mean going to a particular place where you like to meditate, or engaging in an active sport you enjoy.

- Take the performance pressure off yourself. You're the most important person in your world, but you must realize that everyone around you is far too caught up in their own anxieties and issues to notice yours. Remember you don't have to be perfect; be content with being good enough. Be kind to yourself.

It's Not All or Nothing

One of the biggest problems I've seen with people who are excited to start a new healthy eating program is that they have an "all-or-nothing" attitude. They want to get slim overnight and so they quickly become frustrated. When you want to reduce a significant amount of weight, it's easy to fall into all-or-nothing thinking. Unfortunately, this mindset can create a certain air of desperation, which may cause you to rationalize it with arguments similar to these:

- You have to follow a super-strict diet to succeed.
- If you fall off the wagon and eat junk for a day or two, you've blown it altogether so you may as well give up.

This line of thinking can be very detrimental to your weight reduction efforts, but it's easy to fall into that trap. Since how you think about your program is of utmost importance, I've compiled a short list of helpful hints to get your thoughts back on track if you find yourself taking one step forward and three steps back.

Helpful Hint #1: Loosen Up

The first way to avoid all-or-nothing thinking is to shake the idea that you must follow an extremely restrictive diet to reduce your weight. The fact is, most people who successfully manage their weight don't diet at all. They make healthy, permanent lifestyle changes such as cutting back on overall calories, practicing portion control, making better food choices, finding a hobby that gets them outdoors, and reigning in emotional eating. Successful weight reduction focuses on weight management, not just weight reduction.

Helpful Hint #2: Have A Bite Or Two!

Severely limiting your food intake or completely cutting out your favorite foods sets you up to binge. Temptation becomes much less powerful when you can have just a taste of something off limit now and again instead of telling yourself it's off limit for good. This can be difficult at first, but you'll become accustomed to satisfying your cravings with smaller amounts of these tempting foods and learn to enjoy them on occasion in small quantities with just a bite or two.

Helpful Hint #3: Remove The Word "Diet" From Your Vocabulary!

Many people go on and off diets after every holiday season. They say, "I'll start my diet in the New Year," only to be off it by the next weekend. An effective program or lifestyle isn't just to get you ready for the New Year or bikini season; it's to keep you ready for life.

Helpful Hint #4: Forgive Yourself

Let's say you've decided to give Helpful Hint #2 a try and allow yourself your favorite treat: chocolate chip cookies. But you don't stop at a couple…you eat half the package. Then, for breakfast the next morning, you polish off the other half. Have you completely blown it again? Does this mean it's time to give up altogether? Do you think, "Maybe I'm just not cut out for this" and go back to your old eating habits? Absolutely not! Not allowing yourself to make mistakes is the worst error you can make.

Think about this: all-or-nothing thinking is a way to let you off the hook. It's an escape route: "Oh, now I've screwed up. Glad I don't have to bother anymore." There's an old saying that goes, "No matter how far along you are down the wrong path, it's never too late to turn back." So, don't think that just because you made a bad choice today, you can't start over tomorrow, or even later that same day! It sounds like a cliché, but every day, actually every moment, truly is a new beginning. You can't erase last night's binge, but you can aim for a much healthier today!

Helpful Hint #5: Celebrate Small Victories

Praise yourself for the small challenges you surmount; you won't give up so easily if you do. Yes, choosing fish instead of a burger is a victory. Doing an exercise video on Friday is a triumph, even if it's the first day you've exercised this week. Take it easy on yourself as you're learning how to be a new, improved, healthier you. Just don't do it with your feet up!

No matter what health or fitness program you choose, it will be an adjustment for your life. You may not always get it right the first time. Quite often, it's the process of making adjustments that tells you exactly what and how much you need of certain things in your life; think hard about whether you have too much or too little of something. In fact, you may have good reasons why you made the balance tip in a certain direction over time. Have you become tired of your eating regime or exercise routine? Spice it up and beware of boredom! Be honest about what you want and don't want in your life. How important this goal of good health is will shift over time, and that's normal. As long as you're paying attention to your body and living a healthy lifestyle, it's okay to cut back to a couple of times per week at the gym. You don't have to maintain the same regime that helped you get in shape once you're there. Just be sure it doesn't fall by the wayside altogether.

Are You Able And Are You Willing?

Let's take these questions one at a time. Are you able? Are you able to receive, in your physical world, anything you seriously want? It was Napoleon Hill who said that you won't seriously want something that you're not capable of achieving.

"Are you willing?" Are you willing to pay the price that must be paid, realizing there's no such thing as something for nothing. You must create a space for the good that you desire. Everyone's life is full at all times. The question you must ask yourself is, "What is it full of?" Before you can do something else, you must stop whatever it is you're doing and create a space for what you desire.

Are you willing and able to ...

☑ *Make an investment in yourself?*

☑ *Go where you have to go?*

☑ *Do what you have to do?*

☑ *Change what you have to change?*

☑ *Let go of what has to go?*

☑ *Study what must be studied?*

☑ *Take direction when it is required?*

☑ *Continue in the face of failure?*

☑ *Make a 100% commitment to yourself that you'll reach your ideal weight?*

If you checked all the boxes, that's a resounding, "YES – I'M WILLING," so you're already on your way to being at your ideal weight. The material changes must, by natural law, follow.

By following the methods set forth in this book, and the additional information included in *The Complete MindBody FX Lifestyle Program*, you'll not only achieve your ideal weight; you'll gain a new lifestyle that will provide you with a healthy and energetic body and mind. The lessons discussed in this book can be applied to so many areas of your life and will help you with achieving any goal you desire. To learn more and get some delicious and healthy recipes, visit **www.MindBodyFX**. I wish each of you much success with your journey of achieving your ideal weight and living the healthiest, happiest life possible.

Don't Miss Out On Special Bonus #1!!

You already know the information in The MindBody FX Lifestyle will help you achieve your ideal weight, but we want to give you even more assistance to support you on your journey to the life you deserve… for FREE!

Special Report: Tips and Tools for Implementing a Healthier Lifestyle includes invaluable information such as:

✓ Tips for Keeping Control of Serving Sizes

✓ Tips for Family Participation and Support

✓ Tips for Keeping Your Whole Body Happy

✓ Grab and Go Foods

✓ Eating Out Made Easy/Tips for Healthy Eating Out

Download your FREE copy of this very useful report at <u>www.mindbodyfx.com/specialreport1</u>.

Don't Miss Out On Special Bonus #2!!

You already know the information in The MindBody FX Lifestyle will help you achieve your ideal weight, but we want to give you even more assistance to support you on your journey to the life you deserve… for FREE!

Special Report: Toxins and Excess Weight includes invaluable information such as:

✓ What are Toxins?

✓ What's the Link Between Toxins and Weight Loss?

✓ How Toxins are Preventing you from Losing Weight

✓ Toxic Foods, Beauty and Household Products, and Environmental Exposures to Avoid

✓ Tips for Reducing Toxic Exposure

Download your FREE copy of this very useful report at www. mindbodyfx.com/specialreport2.

Don't Miss Out On Special Bonus #3!!

How can you track your success toward achieving your ideal weight? You know from reading The MindBody FX Lifestyle that a scale isn't required, or suggested...but we want to give you a simple way to monitor your progress on your journey to the life you deserve... for FREE!

The Weight Loss Progress Checklist is a great way for you to keep track of:

✓ Your Goal...and the Steps You Need to Take to Reach It

✓ Your Positive Affirmations

✓ New Healthy Eating Habits You're Employing

✓ How Much Water You're Drinking

✓ What Supplements You're Taking

✓ What Changes You Need to Make

✓ What Physical Activities You're Doing

✓ How You'll Reward Yourself for Achieving Mini-Goals

✓ And More!

Download your FREE copy of this very useful checklist at www. mindbodyfx.com/checklist.

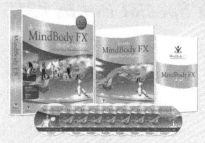
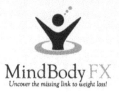

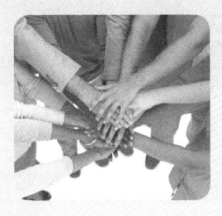

Achieve Success

With Others By Becoming A Support Group Leader

It's very hard, if not impossible, for people to make life changes on their own. You've probably experienced this same feeling before, perhaps with regards to weight loss. In fact, it is the reason we have created our online support tools and forums.

However, we can't support everybody alone... so we're turning to you, because **you have the power to encourage, motivate, and inspire your friends, neighbors, family members to live happier, healthier lives at their ideal weight.**

The MindBody FX Support Group Program Is Already Prepared For You!

We'll provide you with full outlines for conducting each weekly meeting, tools for seeing faster results, and tips for making each get-together a lot of fun!

There's simply no need to struggle on your own or feel like you're all alone ever again!

Please join us in helping others achieve the life they deserve by becoming a Support Group Leader today.

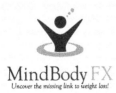

MindBody FX
Uncover the missing link to weight loss!

Visit our web site for more information:
www.MindBodyFX.com

EARN: By signing up for our Affiliate Program at no cost, you can make a commission on any MindBody FX product sales within the group.

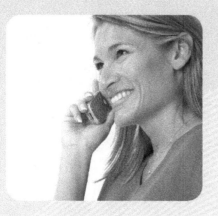
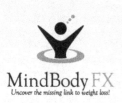

About The Author

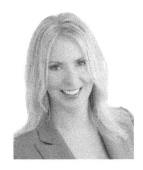

Melonie Dodaro is the founder and CEO of MindBody FX Weight Management Company, the leader in weight loss, specializing in changing the way people think so they can achieve their ideal weight.

Dodaro has a decade of experience owning and operating five weight loss centers throughout the country, in which she helped thousands of clients lose weight and live healthier lives.

She has also worked and studied with many experts in mind potential and human behavior including several of the teachers featured in Rhonda Byrne's "*The Secret*," the acclaimed film that culminates the knowledge from centuries of great thinkers, scientists, artists, and philosophers, on how to live a life of joy and prosperity.

Through her research, Dodaro realized the mind was the missing component in traditional weight loss programs. It's the difference between people achieving their goals, and struggling through life. That's when she developed The MindBody FX Lifestyle to incorporate mental well-being with proven weight loss techniques.

Dodaro now focuses solely on helping people harness the power of their mind to experience the weight loss results they deserve. Her tested and proven MindBody FX programs and products are guaranteed to provide the education and guidance people need to experience healthy, permanent weight loss.

She has certifications in hypnotherapy, Time Line Therapy™, and Neuro-Linguistic Programming (NLP). She is also certified as an NLP master practitioner, motivational coach, life coach, weight loss master coach, and social and emotional intelligence coach.

To find out more about Melonie and The MindBody FX Lifestyle, visit **www.MindBodyFX.com**.

BUY A SHARE OF THE FUTURE IN YOUR COMMUNITY

These certificates make great holiday, graduation and birthday gifts that can be personalized with the recipient's name. The cost of one S.H.A.R.E. or one square foot is $54.17. The personalized certificate is suitable for framing and will state the number of shares purchased and the amount of each share, as well as the recipient's name. The home that you participate in "building" will last for many years and will continue to grow in value.

Here is a sample SHARE certificate:

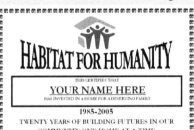

HABITAT FOR HUMANITY

THIS CERTIFIES THAT
YOUR NAME HERE
HAS INVESTED IN A HOME FOR A DESERVING FAMILY

1985-2005
TWENTY YEARS OF BUILDING FUTURES IN OUR
COMMUNITY ONE HOME AT A TIME

1200 SQUARE FOOT HOUSE @ $65,000 = $54.17 PER SQUARE FOOT
This certificate represents a tax deductible donation. It has no cash value.

YES, I WOULD LIKE TO HELP!

I support the work that Habitat for Humanity does and I want to be part of the excitement! As a donor, I will receive periodic updates on your construction activities but, more importantly, I know my gift will help a family in our community realize the dream of homeownership. **I would like to SHARE in your efforts against substandard housing in my community!** *(Please print below)*

PLEASE SEND ME _____ SHARES at $54.17 EACH = $ $_____

In Honor Of: _____

Occasion: (Circle One)   HOLIDAY   BIRTHDAY   ANNIVERSARY

OTHER: _____

Address of Recipient: _____

Gift From: _____ *Donor Address:* _____

Donor Email: _____

I AM ENCLOSING A CHECK FOR $ $_____ PAYABLE TO HABITAT FOR HUMANITY <u>OR</u> PLEASE CHARGE MY VISA OR MASTERCARD *(CIRCLE ONE)*

Card Number _____ Expiration Date: _____

Name as it appears on Credit Card _____ Charge Amount $ _____

Signature _____

Billing Address _____

Telephone # Day _____ Eve _____

PLEASE NOTE: Your contribution is tax-deductible to the fullest extent allowed by law.
Habitat for Humanity • P.O. Box 1443 • Newport News, VA 23601 • 757-596-5553
www.HelpHabitatforHumanity.org

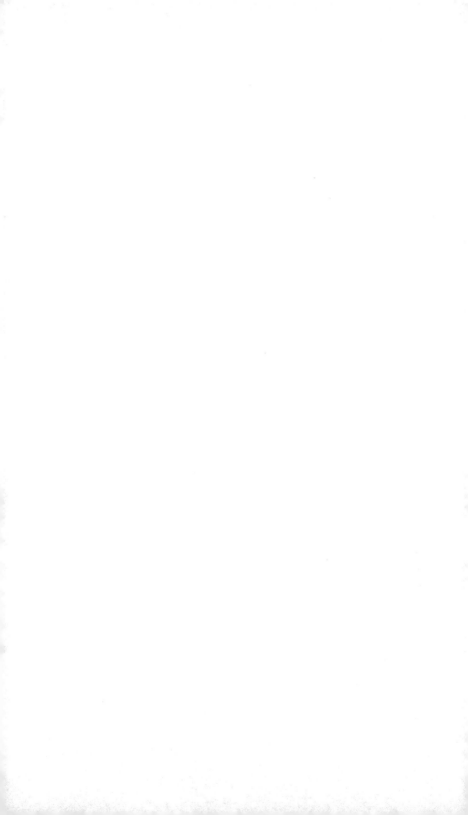